# Finding Genius:
# UNDERSTANDING
# CANCER

### 30 Questions, 70 Geniuses, 200+ Amazing Insights

by **Richard Jacobs, et al**

Edited by: Lindsay Hoeschen

Copyright 2022 by Richard Jacobs, Finding Genius Podcast, Finding Genius Foundation

All rights reserved. No part of this publication may be reproduced, distributed, or transmitted in any form or by any means, including photocopying, recording, or other electronic or mechanical methods, without the prior written permission of the publisher, except in the case of brief quotations embodied in critical reviews and certain other non-commercial uses permitted by copyright law. For permission requests, write to the publisher, addressed "Attention: Permissions Coordinator," at the address below.

Finding Genius Foundation
21750 Hardy Oak Blvd
Suite #104-51700
San Antonio, Texas 78258
www.findinggeniusfoundation.org

Publisher: Finding Genius Foundation, a 501(c)3 Nonprofit

Interviewer and author: Richard Jacobs

Co-Authors: Sandy Bevacqua, Perry Marshall, Mustafa Djamgoz, László Boros, Eric Fung, Jyotsna Batra, Andriy Marusyk, Brendon Coventry, Gábor Balázsi, Henry Heng, Kimberly Bussey, Robert Gatenby, Saverio Gentile, Li Zhang, Jong Bok, Gary Foresman, James Shapiro, George W. Yu, Ben Stanger, Yibin Kang, Xi Huang, Mahmoud Ghannoum, Sendurai Mani, Nathan Crane, Thomas Seyfried, Christos Chinopoulos, Kornelia Polyak, Paul Davies, Jake Becraft, Robert Weinberg, Steven Fiering, Ronald Brown, Doru Paul, Mathew Vander Heiden, Sui Huang, Abdul Kadir Slocum, Adrienne C. Scheck, Ana Soto, Andreas Mershin, Benjamin Hopkins, Carlo Maley, Carlos Sonnenschein, Charley Lineweaver, David Goode, Denis Noble, Dominic D'Agostino, Franois Fuks, George Adrian Calin, Herbert Levine, James DeGregori, Jo Bhakdi, Josh Ofman, Kenneth Pienta, Manel Esteller, Maria Casanova-Acebes, Michael Levin, Patrick S. Moore, Rabia Bhatti, Richard White III, Ruchi Gaba, Samantha Bucktrout, Samuel Sidi, Sandy Borowsky, Seyedtaghi Takyar, Steve Gullans, Steven Eisenberg, Susan Wadia-Ells, William B. Miller

Edited by: Lindsay Hoeschen

Audible audiobook narrated by: Matthew Doyle

Ordering Information:

Quantity sales. Special discounts are available on quantity purchases by corporations, associations, and others. For details, contact the publisher at the address above.

Orders by U.S. trade bookstores and wholesalers.

Please call (888) 988-7381 or visit www.findinggeniusfoundation.org.

Printed in the United States of America

Published January 2022

**ISBN:** 978-1-954506-35-0

# DISCLAIMER

This book is provided for informational purposes only. Do not rely upon the information contained within it to make a medical, health-based, financial, lifestyle, or any other decision. Consult with licensed professionals regarding any health questions or issues you may have. Reading this book does not constitute the practice of medicine, and no doctor-patient relationship is implied nor formed by reading this book.

Many of the co-authors of this book work within the University system; some consult with various corporations, or may seek government or privately-funded grants, and must be extremely careful about their opinions, thoughts, observations, and answers to the questions in this book.

Their words in this book may conflict with the views of some or all of the organizations with which co-authors are involved; readers should not take anything written in this book to be the firm belief of any of the co-authors.

Organizations involved with these co-authors should also understand that the views expressed in this book are to be held completely separate from consideration of their relationships with the co-authors.

All co-authors have been asked to speculate and "let their hair down" in answering these questions to the best of their abilities. They do not claim to be experts based on the questions asked, and specifically disclaim the providing of any advice – this is pure information and speculation.

# DEDICATION

This book is dedication to all those who have suffered from cancer, and to their family members, friends, co-workers, and associates. A cancer diagnoses throws everyone's life into a blender – suddenly your world changes, and death feels like it's just around the corner.

I should know, having faced papillary thyroid cancer myself, and watching my mother pass away from endometrial cancer in April 2020.

Current data says that 50% of all men in the United States and 33% of all women will experience cancer in their lifetimes. This is absurd, and it must not and cannot continue.

There is something terribly wrong with our world when cancer's prevalence is approaching a majority of all human beings. Only death itself, with a 100% occurrence rate, is in the neighborhood of cancer.

Billions upon billions of dollars have been poured into cancer research. Some cancers now have a much higher 5 year survival rate, while many others have no better survival rates than decades ago.

…and no, an extra 3-6 months of life while in a miserable, radiation, surgery, and chemotherapy-ruined state is not "living".

It is my hope that readers will take away potentially useful theories to help others to truly understand cancer, not simply throw another drug at it, or attempt to "trick the body" into stopping cancer.

If you or anyone you know is battling cancer, my heart goes out to you. I know you're thinking about it in the shower, when you wake up, when you lay down to sleep, when someone is talking to you and you're not hearing anything they're saying because your mind is elsewhere. Let's see how we can help.

# Table of Contents

**Introduction** .................................................9
**Part 1 - Cancer: The What, Why and How** ....... 17
What is cancer? ...............................................18
Is cancer a separate life form? ........................21
Is cancer cognitive? .........................................24
What is the difference between a neoplasm,
a benign tumor, and a malignant tumor? .......26
What causes cancer? ......................................29
Viruses that cause cancer ...............................35
What does cancer look like? ..........................38
The structure of a typical solid tumor .............41
The significance of tumor heterogeneity .......43
What abilities and features differentiate cancer
cells from normal cells? ..................................47
The relationship between a tumor's microbiome,
its growth and function ..................................50
What does a cancer cell need to survive? .....53
Today's predominant way of thinking about cancer ......57

**Part 2: The Why** ..................................................................62

Why are some types of cancer more aggressive than others? ...................................................................62

Why and to where do cancers metastasize? ................66

Why might a benign nodule become malignant? ..........70

How cancer ultimately kills ...........................................73

If cancer kills, then why haven't cancer genes been eliminated through natural selection? ....................76

How do cancers behave "primitively"? ........................78

What is the atavistic theory of cancer? ........................81


**Part 3: The How** ...................................................................85

How does cancer first start? ..........................................85

Can cancer start from a single cell? ..............................89

How does cancer metastasize? ......................................92

How do cancer cells communicate and interact with other cells in the body? ..........................................96

Extracellular vesicle production in cancer .....................99

Primary tumor vs metastatic site communication .........102

Evading the host's immune defenses ............................105

Do cancers evolve their own immune system? .............109

How does cancer remission occur? ...............................111

**Part 4: Approaches to Understanding, Detecting, and Treating Cancer** ...... 114

What is missing in our understanding of cancer?.......... 115

Insights from tumor organoid models ............................ 119

Current cancer research projects ................................... 122

**Part 5: Detecting and Diagnosing Cancer** ............... 131

How are most cancers detected and diagnosed today? 131

The benefits of liquid vs. traditional surgical biopsy.... 136

Early detection to improve treatment outcomes .......... 140

**Part 6: Treating Cancer** ............................................. 145

Is the "gold standard" of cancer treatment effective? ..................................................................... 145

Can chemotherapy and/or radiation cause tumor recurrence? ......................................................... 152

How can cancer be treated immunologically? ............. 157

Treating cancer metabolically ...................................... 165

Could the unique microbiome of tumors be used to diagnose or treat cancer? ................................... 178

Emerging, novel approaches to cancer treatment ........ 182

**Co-Author Bios** ........................................................ 193

**References** ................................................................ 282

# INTRODUCTION
## by Richard Jacobs

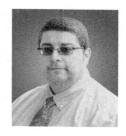

The field of cancer research is massive, all-encompassing, and rapidly expanding. In comparison to other fields and topics on which I have conducted interviews, cancer is, by far, the most complex, diverse, and intensively studied. A search of PubMed alone reveals over 4.3 MILLION scientific papers!

Some might say that to publish a book on cancer without being an oncologist or cancer researcher is ego-filled folly. However, this book contains a wealth of information and conjecture about cancer that is largely missing from many mainstream texts.

The material contained in this book comes from true cancer experts, researchers, clinicians, and brilliant minds – geniuses in the field – no need to rely solely or even significantly upon what I write and think – there's plenty of material here beyond my own opinions.

Just like the old "Hair Club for Men" commercials with Sy Sperling, I'm unfortunately not only a collector and interviewer of cancer experts, but also a "client," having had papillary thyroid cancer myself in 2017. Luckily, I had one of the most favorable cancers you can get –with a 95% five-year survival rate. I didn't have to undergo chemotherapy, although I did have a radical neck dissection (surgery) that took dozens of lymph nodes as well as my thyroid. I also underwent radioactive iodine-131 treatment and watched a series on Chernobyl while isolating at home (yes, my wife yelled at me for watching it, but somehow it was comforting while I was irradiated). One day, if 3D printing of organs is successful, I hope to get a new thyroid... We will see.

Having interviewed over 3,000 researchers, clinicians, CEOs, CSOs, naturopaths, functional medicine doctors, and other super-smart folks, I have a very different perspective on cancer than most.

I believe that to properly understand cancer, it needs to be placed in a radically different framework that emphasizes cellular cognition. Research reveals that cancer behaves as if it was a separate life form. I believe this observation is critical to understanding how cancer starts, why it does what it does, and how to stymie or stop it from killing its host.

No, I'm not saying that cells are as "smart" as people, but cells **do** appear to have their own level of cognition and are incredibly capable of evaluating information, actively adapting to their environment, and have proven successful for 3.8 billion years – if they weren't, none of us would be here to write or read this book!

Call me heretical, but I see the Neo-Darwinist model of random mutation and natural selection as not only severely limited, but nearly completely wrong. My experience of interviewing 3,000+ experts has convinced me that science's view of cancer is missing many critical perspectives, which I describe below.

**Vital perspective #1:** I hypothesize that cancer starts because cells of a given tissue or body system are subjected to chronic, long-term stress (metabolic, chemical, physical, electrical, bacterial, viral, fungal and other exogenous and endogenous stresses) by their nature and biological endowment, cells are able to measure their external and internal micro and macro environment and adapt to stress.

Over time, forced adaptation leads to maladaptation, and triggers cancerous cellular transformation in a tissue or organ, triggering the initiation of an overt cancer. Besides transmissible cancers, this may be how most cancers start.

**Vital perspective #2:** Cells are cognitive.[1] They measure biological information (ex: concentration of a chemical in their microenvironment, the feasibility of trading metabolites with their localized microbiome, their interaction with our immune system, changing expression of various receptors on their cell membranes, generating, releasing, endogenizing and interpreting hundreds of thousands of extracellular vesicles of various types and payloads, etc.) Importantly, cells take contingent action based on these measurements and further analysis by their cellular sensory apparatuses.[1]

Are cells cognitive in the same manner as humans? No. I believe it's unhelpful to compare cells to people in terms of their 'level' of cognition. Cells have different senses than we do as holobionts; cells have different abilities than we do; cells appraise information in a completely alien way than we do. They are not equivalent, or lesser or better, they are simply different, yet capable.

**Vital perspective #3:** Cells have their own senses ("senome"),[2] and their abilities to sense and adapt are different from macroscopic creatures – us, dogs, cows, cats, plants, parasites, etc.

The whole field of epigenetics demonstrates that active adaptation is occurring all the time, at all levels of our body. All living creatures appear to have the ability to modify their DNA or RNA via epigenetic change. Even viruses (which are debated to be alive or not alive) experience epigenetic change during initial infection, latency, endogenization (retroviruses) and subsequent replication and proliferation to additional cellular targets.[3]

In addition, there's a phenomenon known as quorum sensing (thought to be confined to bacteria only, but likely to be a cellular-based ability that extends across all cellular domains and possibly viruses as well) that allows a population of cells to "count" same cell types and "count" other cell types, taking contingent action when measurement of a particular biochemical or cellular entity reaches a certain level.[4-5]

Thanks to my friend, sounding board and brilliant evolutionary biologist, William B. Miller, Jr., I've also learned that biofilms, tissues, organs, and entire organisms are the cellular products of "cellular engineering." Imagine cells wearing little yellow hard hats: cooperating, acting in groups, measuring, coordinating, and orchestrating the creation of biofilms, tissues, organs and organisms.

Cellular engineering puts human engineering to shame. Science can't even reconstitute a single mitochondrion or ribosome, much less a cell, a tissue, an organ, or a living creature. Yet, many scientists have told me that their drug or medical procedure is going to "trick the body" into doing X or Y.

I rarely see scientists including biomimicry or anthropomorphic thinking (highly frowned upon in scientific circles, sadly) in their experimentation or their hypotheses. This makes it dramatically less likely that science will find a 'cure' for cancer or other disorders. This massive underestimation of cellular abilities has delayed and will continue to delay scientific progress for decades to come, in my experience and opinion.

**Vital perspective #4:** Permit yourself the liberty of anthropomorphic reasoning. Unfortunately, nearly every single scientist I've spoken to shies away from deliberate, anthropomorphic analogies in considering biology and evolution. I understand – the entire scientific community, the universities that offer degrees and professorships, the institutions that govern science, and everywhere you look – anthropomorphic thinking is actively frowned upon.

Perhaps this stance should be rethought. Aren't we as humans, collections of trillions of bacteria, viruses, fungi, yeasts, protists, human cells, and more? Without our microbial partners, we would be unable to adequately digest most foods, unable to have robust immune systems, and would literally cease to exist![6] Mitochondria are believed to be bacteria that endogenized into larger cells hundreds of millions of years ago through endosymbiosis. Without mitochondria's cellular capacities, we would never have existed.

The process of endogenization is a salient feature of biology. 8% to 10% of the entire human genome appears to have come from endogenized retroviruses that we were exposed to over evolutionary history?[7] Placental mammals would not exist unless Syncytin (a chemical that allows for the separation of fetus and mother biochemically) endogenized into our DNA long ago.[8]

In addition, humans engage in all the same behaviors that cellular life exemplifies within their interactions in complex cellular ecologies. We engineer, cooperate, coordinate, compete, communicate, reproduce, are born, grow, age and die. So does all life.

If a parasite such as *Toxoplasma gondii* in mice can cause them to not fear cat urine or cats, exposing the mice to a high likelihood of being eaten, allowing this parasite to enter into a different host to complete more of their life cycle,[9] what else are organisms capable of?

How have viruses, which most scientists assume to be inert, non-living entities, successfully infected every living thing for billions of years, adapting and changing in alignment with their infected hosts? Viruses are major drivers of evolution and possibly speciation.[10]

We are composed of many different cellular types (humans, amongst other animals, are superorganisms – aka holobionts). Why do we assume that we're differentially separated from our constituent cells and not ultimately subject to their constraints or privileged by their abilities?

This is why a deliberate inclusion of anthropomorphic thinking is likely to speed along scientific progress and understanding. Don't frown upon it. Embrace it.

**Vital perspective #5:** Cancer appears to represent a different 'self' compared to other cells. The totality of cancer's action, adaption, and self-preservation drive are eerily similar to a separate life form within the larger cellular milieu. Cancer cells should be viewed in part as a separate life form that has all the same proclivities as normal cells plus their own types of idiosyncratic faculties.

Cancer is composed of living things – cells. Cancer is heterogeneous, incredibly adaptive, can reproduce, can 'fool' our immune systems and can spread to foreign tissues.

I hypothesize that cancer becomes a separate life form inside of us. All cells that comprise and compose us must, by definition, be in constant communication with all the other cells and biological entities that comprise us.

Our cells 'talk' to other cells via multiple methods. Our cells 'talk' to our microbiomes and trade metabolites with them. We consume food, which often contains genetic material – it appears that we may be utilizing the genetic material from the food we eat and reacting and adapting to it.[11] Our microbiomes certainly do. Just try changing your diet from keto to vegan or some other significant change and have your microbiome sampled before and after you do. You'll see massive change in terms of which species are present, their prevalence, and hence, the metabolites produced. You'll experience different moods, health, biomarkers, and other changes – some incredibly obvious.

An interview with Florencia McAllister (who studies pancreatic cancer and the pancreatic microbiome – yes, there IS a pancreatic microbiome, not just a gut microbiome)[12] has hugely influenced me by revealing the following:

Cancer tumors are similar to tissues or organs or biofilms in that tumors are comprised of many capable cells that act in concert. These cells communicate and cooperate enough to encourage angiogenesis, possibly use a form of quorum sensing to determine when to metastasize, coordinate action to evade our immune system, and produce specialized extracellular vesicles to communicate with metastatic sites and with our 'healthy cells'.

When attacked by chemotherapy, our immune system, radiation, or other insults, cancer tumors adapt and often recur, in modified form. Instead of being killed by radiation, resection (surgery) or chemotherapy, many cancers adapt and come back more terrible and capable than before, killing their hosts the second or third time around.

Cancer has many of the hallmarks of a separate life form.

Yes, I know many would argue that because cancer often kills its host if not treated, that cancer cannot be a separate life form. At issue is that we don't understand cancer well enough to assert its true aims. What is certain is that cancer learns how to persist in an intelligent, adaptive manner.

As I mentioned above, I hypothesize that cancer **is** a separate life form. Does it start out that way? Is one cancer cell a separate life form, or does this transition happen once sufficient cancer cells are in close proximity?

Life itself appears to be an emergent property of one or more cells; no one can rip apart a person or a cell to find "where the life force is or where the life is." I hypothesize that cells have an individual identity always, whether they are part of a whole, such as our liver cells being a vital part of us as humans, or whether they are single-celled organisms, in biofilms, or in other associations.

Hepatocytes likely 'identify' as hepatocytes, but also as constituents of their localized tissue type in the liver.

Hepatocytes likely have a sense of "self" vs. "other," and also somehow understand that they are part of an organ, and a part of the overarching human as well.

Anthropomorphically speaking, let's say you live in Austin, Texas in the Zilker neighborhood. Are you a Zilkerite? Are you an Austinite? A Texan? A father to two children? A husband, an uncle, an American? Are you a human being? Yes, you are **all** these things. In much the same way, at times, you may consider other people to be family, acquaintances, colleagues, enemies, foreigners, friends, or other constructs.

Cells have their own version of the same phenomenon, and based on which cells have a majority share of 'cellular voice' or resources in a given tissue, a collection of cells may 'identify' as a separate organism – i.e. a cancer tumor, and therefore would have highest allegiance to what they consider to be themselves vs. outsiders.

As you read through this book, I advance the same goal as with the previous Finding Genius Book on viruses. My goal is to produce a speculative, informative, thought-provoking book that will be difficult to outdate or make obsolete for a decade or more.

I urge you to consider the five (5) Vital Perspectives I've outlined above when reading this book, and especially when conducting your own scientific inquiry. My experience of 3,000+ interviews has proven to me many times, that deliberate inclusion of these perspectives will help advance and expedite your scientific inquiry and results.

**Final Note:** This introduction is entirely my own thoughts, assumptions, and assertions. Please do not assume that **any** of the authors share any of my views. As you'll see, most, if not all, have different views than my own.

# PART 1

# CANCER: THE WHAT, WHY, AND HOW

# THE WHAT

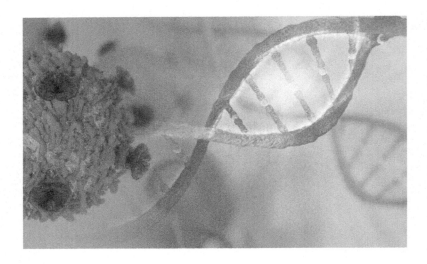

## What is cancer?

**Perry Marshall:**

Cancer is a disease of identity. This isn't something that will be found in most medical textbooks, which is why I believe that traditional approaches are doomed.

Traditional, standard-of-care approaches are never going to work because they rely on the assumption that cancer is just a "disease of the genes," when in reality, the genes are a lagging indicator of cancer cell activity.

**William B. Miller Jr.:**

Cancer is a *verb*. It's about collective cellular actions; Cancer cells co-partner, co-engineer, compete and collaborate in niche construction.

I'd like to plant a seed of thought that cancer is not necessarily a terminus. It's a hard thing for most people to wrap their minds around, but cancer could have a purpose. Why would I say that? Simply because cancer is not random and does not succeed through random actions.

**François Fuks:**

Cancer should be seen as a two-volume book. One volume is well known and has to do with genetic changes (e.g., mutations, chromosomal aberrations), while the other volume—which is likely just as important—has to do with epigenetic changes. Epigenetic changes add a layer of alteration that's often seen in cancer and give way to quite interesting diagnostic and therapeutic applications.

**Saverio Gentile:**

A cancer cell is a cell that has lost control over its proliferation. In other words, it's as though the signals that direct the cell to continue duplicating are always active.

It's important to consider that there is always a balance in nature, and cells are no different. If cells need to proliferate, then there will be signals for proliferation (from one cell comes two, from two comes four, and so on until tissues are organized into organs).

There is an underlying rule that must apply at all times; once proliferation begins, there must be a way for it to stop. For example, cell proliferation must stop at a certain point in order to achieve the necessary size or shape of a particular organ. As another example, cell proliferation is activated when a skin injury is sustained, and stopped once enough cells have surrounded and closed the wound.

Cancer cells use the exact same mechanism of proliferation described in these examples, yet they don't know how to stop proliferating.

**Sandy Borowsky:**

Cancer is not one disease but multiple diseases, and it is initiated with an intrinsic set of abilities. In addition to that set of abilities, cancer will grow only if and when it encounters the right opportunities and the right environment.

Each initiated cancer is somewhat unique, but there are commonalities related to the cell of origin. There are about 100 different specialized cells that make up breast tissue, and at least one subset of those is susceptible to becoming cancer. Depending on which of those cells is initiated, there are different potential outcomes.

However, those potential outcomes won't occur unless certain conditions are met within the environment and the host's immune system, much of which is regulated by the host's health, nutrition, microbiome, and genetics. The outcome can be the result of a complicated interaction that involves the initiation of a specific type of cancer from a specific cell, along with a constellation of environmental cues or miscues.

**Paul Davies:**

Cancer is immensely complex, isn't it? The job of a cosmologist and theoretical physicist is to look through the complexity and try to boil things down to the deep, underlying principles.

On the one hand, cancer looks very complicated and differs from patient to patient. On the other hand, it looks very systematic and highly organized, almost as if there's a blueprint or plan of action that is followed by most cancers in most organisms.

# Is cancer a separate life form?

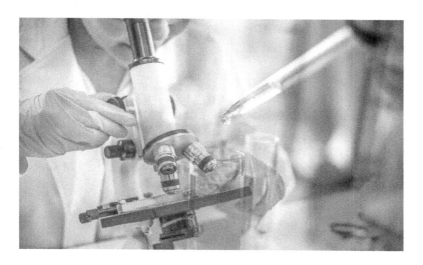

**James DeGregori:**

In 99.9% of cases, cancer is not a separate organism because it dies with the host, which means it is terminal for itself as well. However, there are rare exceptions, such as devil facial tumor disease (DFTD) in Tasmanian devils, venereal tumors in dogs, and leukemia in clams. These cancers are actually spread from individual to individual.

In Tasmania, there are two cancers that are almost eliminating the Tasmanian devil population, although the latest news is that Tasmanian devils are starting to become resistant and the population may survive.[13] The original venereal dog tumor originated in a dog thousands of years ago, and that single transformational event has spread throughout the globe in thousands of other dogs.[14]

In these rare cases, cancer essentially becomes its own organism. In the vast majority of cases, however, cancer is very much dependent on the host for growth factors and overall survival. When cancer cells are removed from a host, they will die if not cultured with the resources they would normally receive from the host. Therefore, they're certainly not independent entities.

**Sui Huang:**

It's a bit eerie to think of cancer as a separate life form. Like any disease, cancer is a reconfiguration of the mechanisms that make us strong and robust, but it's reconfigured in a maladaptive way. It takes advantage of many biological processes that we need in order to stay alive, and in that sense, cancer is like a separate life form.

**Henry Heng:**

To answer this question, we need to step back and define cancer. Traditionally, cancer has been defined as a disease of the cell that occurs via uncontrolled cell proliferation and other features of growth (e.g., evading cell death pathways, escaping the immune system, etc.).

However, through a series of macro-evolutionary events, a completely different karyotype (i.e., complete set of chromosomes of a species or organism) has emerged. Distinct biological systems have different karyotypical coding systems, and cancer meets this definition.[15] Accordingly, we need to think of cancer as a new cellular system that emerged from normal tissue and is genetically quite different from the host cell.

From this perspective, we certainly support the idea that cancer is a new cellular species. Of course, this is a very provocative idea that some will find hard to accept.

In addition, treatment-induced genome reorganization represents a novel mechanism for drug-induced rapid drug resistance in cancer". This message is of importance to search for new strategies for cancer treatment.[267]

**Saverio Gentile:**

In short, no. Cancer is really nothing more than a normal cell that has a different way of controlling certain parameters. One of the problems is that often we don't know how a normal cell behaves…

**Steven Fiering:**

It's almost philosophical, but I think of cancer as being a parasite, feeding off the host to the detriment of the host. At the same time, cancer has its own goal; its programming is such that it is going to divide and ignore the signals that tell it not to divide, and it's going to continue taking resources from the host until the degradation of that host.

# Is cancer cognitive?

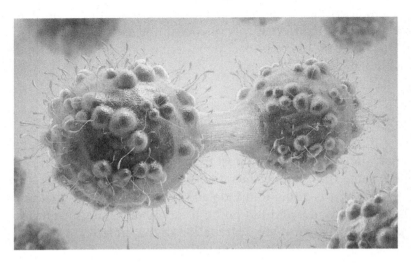

**Perry Marshall:**

Cells, by any reasonable definition, are smart. They do not evolve accidentally through simple random mutation and natural selection; they evolve smartly, actively participate in their own evolution, and make educated guesses about what responses will work best in a given context.

In late-stage cancers, the cancer cells are collectively smarter than every doctor and every scientist. The fundamental mistake of evolutionary biology is the assumption that cells are dumber than we are. In truth, they are smarter than us—we just don't know by how much.

**Sui Huang:**

Cancer cells are very complex, and very often we mistake complexity for evidence of cognition. There are computer programs that allow the user to invent cells and endow them with certain properties, and I think that's probably what's going on. In other words, it looks like cancer cells have a mind of their own, but in reality, they don't.

**William Miller Jr:**

Cancer cells are cognitive agents that deal with ambiguous, imprecise, and uncertain information, yet manage to find little cues in cellular environments. Cancer has its own form of creativity, but ordinary researchers have not concentrated on this.

Cancer is a form of cognitive entanglement with its cellular milieu, yet cancer research is still imbued with Darwinism and Neo-Darwinism (i.e., randomness, purposelessness). What I am proposing is an antonym for Neo-Darwinism; I'm saying we need to look at cancer beyond Neo-Darwinism, on the basis of the *intelligent* measuring cell.

# What is the difference between a neoplasm, a benign tumor, and a malignant tumor?

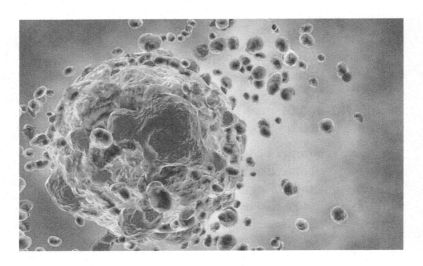

**Brendon Coventry:**

The term 'neoplasm' is often used interchangeably with the term 'cancer,' but neoplasm simply means new cell growth (neo = new, plasm= forming cells) and a neoplasm can be benign or malignant.

In general, benign tumors have a pushing border which grows outwardly in a more orderly way than malignant tumors, which tend to have an invasive border. Malignant tumors can also be surrounded by a pseudo capsule, as well as a pushing border.

There are many types of tissues that are regarded as benign but behave in a very malignant way. One such example is the mammalian placenta.[16]

**Jo Bhakdi:**

Neoplasms form from the abnormal growth of cells, and they can be benign or malignant. Both benign and malignant neoplasms are referred to as tumors.

Benign tumors might grow, but won't spread throughout the body (i.e., metastasize) and therefore generally won't create problems. However, a tumor at any place in the body can be surprisingly dangerous if it grows uncontrollably, even if it does not metastasize.

It is the ability to metastasize that makes a tumor malignant.

**Doru Paul:**

Since a neoplasm is just an area of new tissue growth, which can be benign or malignant, this question is really about the difference between benign tumors and malignant tumors.

The primary difference between benign tumors and malignant tumors is that benign tumors don't break membranes, do not invade locally, and do not spread to distant parts of the body. Since the description of Warburg of the aerobic glycolysis in the '30s, we know that metabolic changes play a key role in the inception of malignant tumors but not of benign tumors. So, at the cellular level, there are genetic, epigenetic and metabolic differences between benign and malignant tumors.

Genetic mutations cannot always differentiate between a benign tumor and a malignant tumor. As an example, mutations of the BRAF gene can be found in both benign tumors and melanoma,[17] an aggressive type of skin cancer, which suggests, that at the genetic level, some benign and malignant tumors may be very similar. For malignant tumors to occur, besides genetic alterations, epigenetic factors also play an important role. An important point to remember: zooming out, cancer is not solely a disease of the cell, it is also a stromal disease, and, as I have shown in "The systemic hallmarks of cancer", a disease of the whole organism.

**Saverio Gentile:**

A tumor is just a cellular mass and is not necessarily dangerous, meaning that it won't necessarily moves around (metastasize) or disrupt the tissue from which it stems.

In contrast, malignant growth is uncontrolled and doesn't follow specific rules in terms of interacting directly with the surrounding tissue. As a result, the tendency of a malignant tumor is to disrupt and destroy the surrounding tissue.

On top of that, a malignant tumor can become metastatic, meaning cells from the primary tumor can shed, moves, invade the bloodstream, and eventually end up in other body compartments where it will proliferate and form another mass. Often, if proliferation is the main cancer character, metastasis is the real clinical problem.

**Christos Chinopoulos:**

Neoplasms can be benign or metastatic. A benign neoplasm will be well encapsulated, and the cells will demonstrate contact inhibition.19 This means that several benign neoplastic cells placed next to one another will not begin proliferating, even after contact with one another.

In contrast, metastatic cells will proliferate on one another and create many layers of additional cells, which will eventually spread to different organs. In addition, metastatic tumors have organ predilections (e.g., the tendency to go from the lung to the brain, or from the liver to the lung).

# What causes cancer?

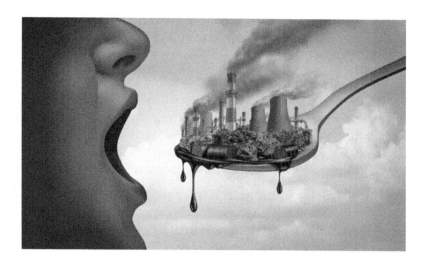

**Nathan Crane:**

Once people learn what actually causes cancer and what can be done to prevent and reverse it, they won't have to be afraid of it anymore. Most people just don't understand these things, and unfortunately, neither do most medical professionals. This includes oncologists, who simply aren't trained in cancer causation, prevention, or healing; they are trained in surgery, pharmacology, chemotherapy, and radiation.

There is a consortium of different causes of cancer, including poor diet (e.g., dairy, meat and processed food), toxins in the food, water, body-care products and air, lack of physical activity, chronic stress, and negative emotional states. We also know that anything that causes DNA damage (e.g., carcinogens) can lead to cancer cell creation in the body.[20]

Carcinogens are everywhere, including the food we eat, the water we drink, the products we put on our bodies (e.g., makeup, lotion, deodorant), the exhaust coming from our cars, and the volatile organic compounds (VOCs) emanating from our carpets, painted walls, etc.[21-22] When these toxins enter the body, they cause DNA damage, which causes cells to enter a chronically fermentative state in order to survive. If the body cannot get rid of these cells fast enough, they can become cancerous.

One of the first things people need to understand is that cancer is inside each and every one of us; it's inside me and it's inside every person who is reading this right now. But we are all equipped with an immune system that is designed to identify and eliminate cancer cells from the body before they multiply and form a cancerous tumor.

This begs the question: Why will almost 50% of the global population be diagnosed with cancer at some point in their lives, and why do approximately 10 million people worldwide die every year from cancer[23] and its treatments?

It's because our immune systems are not fully functioning, which is because they are being inhibited every single day as a result of our diet, lifestyle, environment, and mindset.

The bottom line is this: For as long as a person has a fully functioning immune system, they will not receive a cancer diagnosis. Dozens of integrative medical doctors around the world echo this exact statement.

**James DeGregori:**

What *prevents* us from getting cancer? That's the other side of this question, and the answer is a normal environment.

As a species, we evolved *not* to get cancer—at least not until after the reproductive years. This is because the goal of natural selection is to maximize reproductive success, which requires fit bodies that are unlikely to die from intrinsic reasons during the period of time when passing on genes is most likely.

This provides an explanation for why we avoid cancer quite well. We have trillions of cells and we're loaded with oncogenic mutations, but we rarely get cancer in the first half century of life; this is quite a feat, possible only by virtue of the body's ability to keep these mutations in check.

This line of reasoning leads to the argument that the normal tissue environment favors the normal phenotype, and if that tissue environment is perturbed, it will favor a different—or even malignant—phenotype. In other words, malignant evolution is promoted by an altered environment.[24,71]

The alterations could be caused by aged tissues during the post-reproductive period. Other causes might be related to lifestyle. For example, smoking perturbs the lung environment to such a degree that a stem cell in the lungs of a smoker is in an environment that differs greatly from the environment intended by evolution. As a result, there will be pressure on the lung cells of a smoker to adapt to the new environment, and through that adaptation, a malignant phenotype could be favored.

**Susan Wadia-Ells:**

Thomas Seyfried's ground-breaking research, described in his 2012 text, Cancer as a Metabolic Disease: On the Origin, Management and Prevention of Cancer, has shown that the origin of a person's first cancer cell is caused by the suffocation of that cell's mitochondria[25]—the batteries of the cell.

There are many lifestyles and life experiences that can suffocate a breast cell's mitochondria. For example, an overweight woman's excess fat cells constantly produce a weak form of estrogen, creating a toxic excess of estrogen that enters a woman's breast cells.[26] Once there, it can contribute to the suffocation of the cells' mitochondria and initiate the development of cancer in the breast.

**Ronald Brown:**

A focus of my research has been on the connection between phosphate toxicity and tumorigenesis.

Adults need about 700 milligrams of phosphorus per day, which is an essential micronutrient. If phosphorus intake becomes too high for the kidneys to sufficiently regulate, then it can start accumulating in the body. The accumulation of phosphorus can cause phosphate toxicity, which can affect every organ system in the body and cause death in a short period of time.

Phosphorus also stimulates growth. Consider fertilizers: They are used to stimulate growth in plants, and one of the most common ingredients is phosphorus.[27] In fact, extensive use of phosphorus-containing fertilizers has caused eutrophication, a process whereby phosphorus begins to accumulate in bodies of water where it feeds the growth of algae, leading to harmful algae blooms.[28] This process is due to the fact that phosphorous stimulates growth.

Evidence shows that the same process can occur in the human body, where phosphate toxicity promotes tumor cell growth.[29] The body stores excess phosphorus in solid tumor sites in order to keep it out of circulation, thereby preventing phosphate toxicity. There is a reciprocal relationship between phosphorus and cancer cell growth: Phosphorus stimulates the growth of the cell, and that additional growth becomes the tumor, which helps sequester more phosphorus.

My research is aimed at identifying how to prevent excess phosphorus from getting into our bodies in the first place; I argue that a high phosphorus diet is likely the most modifiable cause of cancer that we can control.

**Thomas Seyfried:**

Many people say that the cause of cancer is always genetic. For example, mutations in the BRCA1 and BRCA2 genes are pointed to as the cause of breast cancer. But interestingly, these mutations will only cause cancer if they damage mitochondria; 40% - 50% of women who have the BRCA1 or BRCA2 mutation never develop breast cancer[30] because—for whatever reason—the mutation does not damage mitochondrial respiration.

There are many provocative agents that can cause cancer. Nobel laureate, Albert Szent-Györgyi, referred to the oncogenic paradox, which is the idea that cancer can be caused by almost anything.[31] X-rays are just one example; we know they damage the respiratory process of oxidative phosphorylation in mitochondria,[32] which can cause intermittent hypoxia (low oxygen levels) and inflammation in an organ. The result is compensatory fermentation and the path to unbridled proliferation—the initiation of a tumor.

Once we know how to connect the dots, it's not all that complicated.

**Gábor Balázsi:**

Molecular causes and mechanisms of cancer comprise an infinite field. People are discovering an increasing number of these mechanisms, which besides genetic mutations include epigenetic changes (e.g., histone acetylation, DNA methylation). These chemical modifications are being investigated by a number of emerging single-cell analysis tools and are being described in detail.

However, I'd like to emphasize that there are other important mechanisms which can cause cancer, such as positive feedback. Positive feedback does not necessarily require any particular chemical modification mechanism except a gene activating itself to increase its protein production, which fuels even more protein production.33 In other words, a gene makes a protein that activates protein synthesis from that same gene.

When this happens, either directly or indirectly, it can lead to states where initially identical cells can diverge and sustain either a high protein level or low protein level. This self-sustaining cycle can lead to a somatically heritable, non-genetic change that is not tied to any specific epigenetic mechanism. This is a topic that pervades all of biology; it's not specific to cancer.

# Viruses that cause cancer

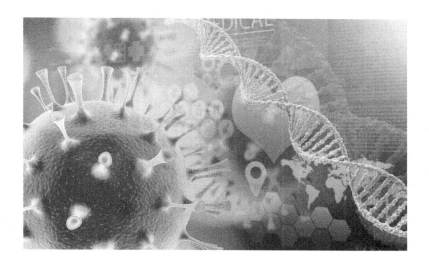

**Robert Gatenby:**

Human papillomavirus (HPV) is a great example of a virus that is causative of cancer.[40] HPV enters and takes over much of the machinery of the cell for the purposes of the virus, but things can go awry, resulting in the formation of a cancer cell.

The conventional wisdom is that 10% - 20% of cancers are caused by viruses,[41] but people who study this tend to think this is a significant underestimate.

**William Miller Jr.:**

I do not believe that the mechanism by which a virus turns a normal cell into a cancer cell is known. A solid association between viruses and cancers has been identified, but if a virologist were asked to explain the exact mechanism behind this association, I don't think they'd be able to.

**Patrick Moore:**

The field of cancer research has gone back and forth multiple times in terms of whether viruses cause cancer. It began around 1909 with a discovery by Peyton Rous of a virus that causes cancer in chickens.[34] It was clear that transmission of this virus to chickens would cause cancer, but for decades following that discovery, no one was able to show in humans or other mammals that viral transmission causes cancer.

Interest in the idea that viruses cause cancer wasn't piqued again until the 1950s and early 1960s, when a number of cancer-causing viruses were found in rodents.[35-37] What followed was an enormous burst of enthusiasm for finding viruses as the fundamental cause not just of *some* cancers, but *all* cancers.

The Epstein-Barr virus (EBV) was the first to be identified as a cancer-causing virus in humans.[38] This discovery began in 1964, when an Irish surgeon by the name of Denis Parsons Burkitt identified a pediatric cancer (now known as Burkitt lymphoma) while in Africa. Noticing that this cancer was markedly different than those he had studied in Europe, he brought back a sample to his laboratory in England, where Tony Epstein and Yvette Barr worked as his graduate students.

A very quality electron microscope image of the cultures revealed the presence of a virus—a type of herpesvirus now referred to as Epstein-Barr virus. From that point forward, scientists have declared that, indeed, this virus causes cancer. However, it isn't entirely clear *how* or *why* it causes cancer. In fact, Epstein-Barr virus is a rather ubiquitous infection, with which at least 95% of healthy adults are infected.[39]

**Steven Fiering:**

There are many well-known viruses that manipulate oncogenes and tumor suppressor genes, such human papilloma virus, that causes most cervical cancers. Other human viruses also cause cancer, such as Epstein-Barr Virus. An early virus identified as causing cancer in monkeys is SV40. SV40 is known to express large T antigen, which is a protein that interferes with tumor suppressor genes and causes changes that can lead to cancer.[42]


**Richard A. White III:**

There is a litany of tumor-causing viruses. In fact, viruses are actually used to create immortalized cells and cell lines.[43-44] It's been estimated that 17.8% of all human cancers are caused by infection, whereas 11.9% are caused by viruses.[45]

Some of the heavy-hitter oncoviruses include the following:

1. Epstein–Barr virus.[38]
2. Hepatitis C virus, which can cause hepatocellular carcinoma.[46]
3. Human T-cell leukemia/lymphoma virus (HTLV-1 and HTLV-2). Originally, HIV was called HTLV-3, until it was found to cause another disease—AIDS.[47] The other type of cancer that is associated with HIV is Kaposi sarcoma-associated herpesvirus (KSHV).[48] When people have severe autoimmunity issues due to HIV, Kaposi sarcoma shows up and causes large blotches all over the body.
4. Adenoviruses can induce cancer in rodents.[49]
5. Human papillomavirus (HPV), for which there is now a vaccine, can cause several types of cancer, including head and neck cancer.[40]
6. Simian virus 40 (SV40) can cause tumors in rodent models, but it is not believed to be oncogenic in humans.[50]

# What does cancer look like?

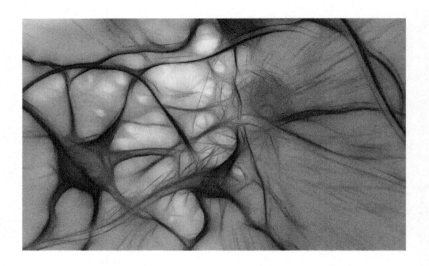

**Sandy Borowsky:**

A cell that is spending all of its energy on DNA replication will have a higher nuclear-to-cytoplasmic ratio as opposed to a cell carrying out more normal activities, such as protein production in the cytoplasm. This is because the nucleus is the site of DNA replication, whereas protein-related activities of the cell occur in the cytoplasm.

As a cell becomes more geared toward replication (as in the case of a cancer cell), the nuclear-to-cytoplasmic ratio will increase, and this can be observed microscopically.[51] When the ratio between the size of the nucleus and cytoplasm of a cell is high, it indicates that the cell has forgotten how to function as a normal cell, and also points to a higher grade of cancer.

The counterexample to this is that there are instances where cells become very large during a reactive process to abnormal stimuli. For example, when a normal cell reacts to an injury caused by radiation, both the nucleus and cytoplasm will enlarge as the cell works harder to do what a normal cell does in response to an injury.

**George Yu:**

The shape of a cancer cell on light microscopy H & E stain is obvious in that the shape is not uniform and the Nucleus is bigger and darker and at times we see dividing cells in fast growing cancers like testicular cancer. With electron microscopy which has a much higher magnification, you start seeing very abnormal organelles such as the mitochondria which is the cigar-shaped energy factory within normal cell. In 1978 Doctor Peter Pedersen, one of my mentors at Johns Hopkins showed me that cancer mitochondria had many different shapes and the more aggressive the cancer, the fewer mitochondrial organelles within the cell. He also noted the cell membrane had a different ratio of cholesterol to phosphatidylcholine molecules, thus changing its function and shape.

**Rabia Bhatti:**

The appearance of a tumor will depend on the stage of cancer. At the early stage, we may not see anything with the naked eye, but microscopically we will see fibrous strands and cancer cells running through the tissue.

When resecting a high-grade tumor, I can usually feel hard and gritty tissue under my knife; this is how I know that I need to remove extra tissue to ensure I get clear margins.

**Dominic D'Agostino:**

Since tumor cells don't talk to one another in the same way normal cells in normal tissues talk to one another, there is no elegant, coordinated structure to the blood vessels within a tumor. Instead, they appear erratic and disorganized.

**Ana Soto:**

The majority of cancers are not just amorphous blobs; they look like the tissue of origin, with some deviations. Depending on the type of tumor, there may be a visible separation between the tumor and normal tissues; no such separation can be seen in the case of invasive tumors.

# The structure of a typical solid tumor

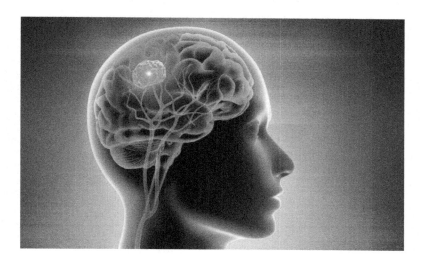

**Denis Noble:**

There are two things worth noting with regard to the structure of a typical solid tumor. First, exosomes are involved in "preparing the way" for a metastatic process by actually placing what one might call 'sticky' proteins on the path.[54]

Second, angiogenesis (i.e., the development of new blood vessels) is a part of the structure. If a cancerous tissue develops without a blood supply, it will die. To remain alive indefinitely, the tissues must be within a few hundred microns of circulating fluid. Thus, in order to survive, cancerous tissues must promote the necessary circulation.[53]

**Seyedtaghi Takyar:**

As a tumor grows, the cells in the center of the tumor die, creating what's referred to as a necrotic center.[53] This cell death occurs because the tumor has improper tissue organization, which prevents proper formation of blood vessels. As a result, blood cannot be sent to the center of the tumor, and the cells die.

This is one of the major differences between a tumor and an organ; an organ enlarges (to a degree) and has vascularity at every single level, whereas a tumor enlarges but does not have vascularity at every level.

**Christos Chinopoulos:**

A metastatic solid tumor that grows very fast will have a necrotic center surrounded by a penumbra region that is hyperperfused, but metabolically extremely active. Most of the cells responsible for the clonality of cancers reside in this penumbra area.

Outside the penumbra is a layer of cells that form the stroma, employ fibroblasts on the nearby normal tissue to feed the cancer cells, induce angiogenesis, and become 'immunologically blank' (i.e., undetectable by the host's immune system).

**Gábor Balázsi:**

The structure of a tumor depends on which stage of growth it is in, as well as how far it is from the baseline of normal epithelia. During tumor growth, the middle of the tumor becomes hypoxic, which incentivizes migration, while the exterior has access to supplies which allow it to continue growing.[53]

When cells begin migrating away from this structure, they respond to their environment and develop more heterogeneity. In essence, there will be the village, and the herd of vagabonds around it.

When metastasis is formed, this whole process is reinitiated, meaning that a vagabond cell (which could initially be dormant), will start growing, and eventually form a tumor that will develop a hypoxic interior, an actively growing exterior, and another herd of vagabond cells migrating away.

# The significance of tumor heterogeneity

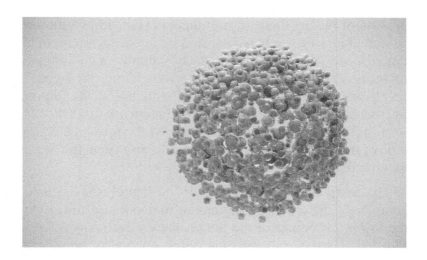

**Kenneth Pienta:**

As cancer cells mutate, they create many different kinds of clones, which leads to tumor cell heterogeneity. If one were to look at a billion cancer cells, they'd be able to determine that they came from the same parent cell, but just like children, they would all look slightly different, and each would have different abilities in terms of growth rate, secretions, invasion, etc.

There is also host cell heterogeneity, which refers to various white blood cells (e.g., T cells, macrophages, dendritic cells, neutrophils, basophils), stromal cells (e.g., fibroblasts), and organ cells (e.g., prostate cells, ductal cells, liver cells, etc.).

In response to the presence of cancer, each type of cell will react differently in terms of reforming the tumor microenvironment.[55] At any given time, there are about 30 different cell types carrying out difference activities, depending on the microenvironment.

**Jo Bhakdi:**

Tumor heterogeneity primarily refers to the mutational profiles of the hundreds of millions of cells within a tumor. In one study, researchers biopsied different locations of a tumor, and then barcoded each sample with unique molecular identifiers.[56] Once they were done, they could reverse-engineer the 3D mutational structure of the tumor. In essence, this means that they could sequence 10,000 cells from different locations, which allowed them to locate any type of mutation as a percentage of cells from specific areas of a tumor.

By analyzing the 3D tumor structure, they found completely different populations of mutational profiles: At the lower left corner of the tumor, there were many KRAS (Ki-ras2 Kirsten rat sarcoma viral oncogene homolog) mutations, and on the upper right corner of the tumor, there were no KRAS mutations. Further, one side of the tumor had a much lower frequency of mutation in the gene for EGFR (epidermal growth factor receptor) than the other side.

These findings were actually very disturbing, because the assumption of current oncology is that one sample of a tumor is representative of the entire tumor, and that therapy can be chosen based upon the sequencing data of one sample.

Making that assumption is like entering a village full of terrorists, taking a picture of one terrorist, and assuming that all of the other terrorists look exactly the same. Even if there are 10 terrorists who indeed look exactly the same as the terrorist in the photo, there are countless other terrorists in the village that will remain unaccounted for. In fact, taking out those 10 terrorists would make the other terrorists stronger because it would leave them with less competition.

## Xi Huang:

Our work suggests that mechanical heterogeneity is a very important physical trait in cancer. We found that depending on the geographical location of the measurement point, local tissue stiffness within the same tumor can vary greatly[57]. In some regions within medulloblastoma, which is the most common pediatric malignant brain tumor, tissue stiffness is comparable to that in non-tumor brain regions, but in other regions of the same tumor, stiffness can be 10 to 20 times greater.

We believe this difference in tissue stiffness can translate to geographically different cancer cell behaviors, malignancy states, and therapy responses. How do tumor cells residing in different places sense and respond to tissue stiffness heterogeneity? Hopefully we will have an answer to that question within the next couple of years.

## Kornelia Polyak:

What drives evolution? Heterogeneity, selection, and reproduction—and the same can be said about tumor development. If tumors were not heterogeneous, then they would be homogeneous, and therefore curable with the use of a single drug.

As the cell population within a tumor grows, there is regeneration of a different type of heterogeneity, and this regeneration—this process of evolution—occurs over and over as a tumor develops. Evolution is very hard to stop, which is why it is so difficult to treat advanced-stage and recurrent tumors.

The three drivers of progression are heterogeneity, selection, and proliferation; modulating any one of them (or all three, ideally) is the most effective way to control cancer.

It can be beneficial to inhibit or slow cell proliferation, even if it is not stopped altogether.

When it comes to metastatic disease, heterogeneity increases as a result of tumor growth in different places in the body.[58] For instance, a tumor that's located in the brain encounters a completely different environment than a tumor that's located in the lung. The cancer cells that can survive in the given environment will be strongly selected for, which means each metastatic site will be composed of cells exhibiting different abilities in accordance with the particular microenvironment. Overall, this creates a higher level of heterogeneity.

# What abilities and features differentiate cancer cells from normal cells?

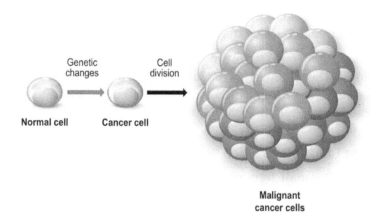

Malignant cancer cells

**Dominic D'Agostino:**

I would say that the initial step in oncogenic transformation is self-sufficiency in growth signals. A cancer cell just wants to become autonomous and return to an archaic form where it is insensitive to anti-growth signals. This indels the cancer cell with unbridled proliferation, and it becomes almost separate from the body; it walls itself off, creates various proteins and glycoproteins, and can become resistant to the immune system.

**William Miller Jr.:**

Cancer cells use cellular tools in a different way than normal cells do. For instance, cancer cells—unlike normal cells—can go backwards in their toolbox; it's like reverse evolution; not only do they have the differentiated skills of a normal modern cell, but for reasons that we don't understand, they can turn backwards and call upon profound survival mechanisms that are part of a huge, long evolutionary learning curve.

Cancer cells can deploy these mechanisms in ways that regular cells cannot, which results in a different life cycle, absence of apoptosis, and immortal clonal lineages, all of which are features that distinguish them from normal cells.

This means that cancer can find solutions to cellular ecological problems by securing cellular resources and outcompeting normal cells. And it can do all of these things because it is a self-referential, measuring, intelligent agent.

**Steven Fiering:**

Likely, one of the first abilities a normal cell acquires on its way to becoming a cancer cell is proliferation despite regulatory signals to cease proliferation. Rather than developing into a well-behaved benign tumor, proliferation continues, and mutations and epigenetic changes accumulate. As a result, the tumor becomes potentially recognizable by the immune system, at which point it may begin to develop a resistance mechanism against the immune system. Another feature of cancer cells is expression of telomerase that modifies the ends of chromosomes and is required to make cancer cells able to divide indefinitely.

**Gábor Balázsi:**

The most important ability of a cancer cell is to grow without the appropriate signal. When it comes to breast cancer, most are estrogen receptor (ER) positive, which means an active estrogen receptor overreacts to signals for cell growth. Typically, this growth occurs at a normal rate, but when the estrogen receptor is overexpressed, growth occurs at a much higher rate, and even irrelevant, small signals may cause the cells to proliferate.[59]

The other side of this coin is that abnormal (e.g., infected, injured, abnormally proliferating) cells in the body are required to die via programmed cell death (i.e., apoptosis); despite being abnormal, cancer cells can evade death.[60]

Both the ability to grow without the appropriate signal and the ability to evade death confer advantages to cancer cells.

# The relationship between a tumor's microbiome, its growth and function

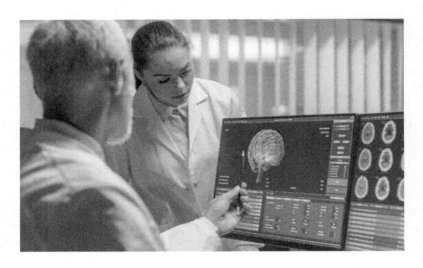

**Saverio Gentile:**

The microbiome can be permissive for cancer to develop, but it can also be suppressive by interfering with tumor growth.[61-62] This interference is not necessarily physical in nature—like breaking the defensive lines in football—but chemical. Some microbiomes secrete collections of chemicals that the cancer cells use for growth, while others secrete collections of chemicals that inhibit tumor growth.

Certain types of bacteria can even indicate the presence of a tumor, which is just one tool at the disposal of clinicians in detecting cancer.[61]

**Dominic D'Agostino:**

The microbiome is responsible for making an entire cascade of things, including serotonin and various inflammatory factors that can influence tumor growth and invasiveness by not only expanding the biomass of a tumor, but influencing the microenvironment.[61]

A tumor that exists within a particular organ can change the entire microbiome of that particular organ, which can then produce epigenetic changes that can further alter and influence the metastatic cascade.

This topic is on the fringe of what most people are studying now, but several papers have been published detailing the ways in which tumors affect the microbiome of different organs.

**Carlo Maley:**

If cancer cells produce different microbial metabolites, then they produce a microenvironment that selects for microbes that are good at living in that environment; in turn, the microbial metabolites change the environment and the selective pressures on tumors.

This leads to a prediction that Athena Aktipis and I made, which is that some microbes are particularly well-adapted to cancerous or precancerous tissue, and are under selection to promote the growth of that tissue.[63] In this way, cancerous or precancerous growths may be driven in part by the microbes that benefit from the microenvironment.

This may be particularly likely in some colorectal cancers, as well as the precancerous state referred to as Barrett's esophagus. In the latter, there is a cryptlike architecture that appears as small wells or incubators where bacteria can grow.[64] People don't really think of these wells as incubators, but as a way of increasing the surface area for absorption of liquids. Regardless, they are niches for the growth of microbes. And if there is a mutant or precancerous niche, then there would be selection for the microbes to create additional crypts, thereby providing a greater environment for cancerous growth.

**Mahmoud Ghannoum:**

Several epidemiological studies have looked at the relationship between poor oral hygiene and tumorigenesis in the mouth. Findings show that in people who have poor oral hygiene and resultant dysbiosis (an imbalance of microbes in the mouth), the incidence of tumorigenesis is higher—not only in the mouth, but in the gut, lung, and other parts of the body.[65]

**Robert Gatenby:**

The problem is that we keep making observations about the relationship between the microbiome and tumors without any good theory to back them up.

Let's assume the microbiome affects the development of colon cancer, which would make perfect sense. But how does that happen? And how does the tumor change the microbiome? What specific factors draw a line from one dot to the next?

These questions give rise to a more general problem involving the microbiome: It can change overnight, and it can differ even within a single organ. Just as our diet can change on a day-to-day basis, the microbiome can too.

It is difficult to track down the effects of something that's always in flux, and to connect these changes with tumours that are equally dynamic. This is especially true since a tumor could be exposed to a large number of microbiomes over the course of several years. Ultimately, we need a consistent theory to put together all of the factors involved.

# What does a cancer cell need to survive?

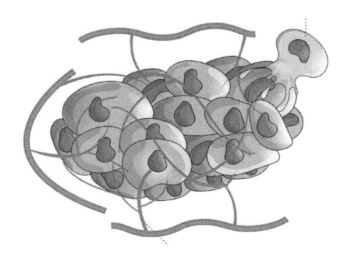

**Thomas Seyfried:**

It's important to understand that all cancers are the same, whether it's brain, colon, or breast cancer. They all have the same underlying problem, which is the inability to use oxygen to generate energy. As a result, they use fermentation to generate energy.[66]

There are only two major fuels that drive fermentation: glucose and glutamine. This means that if glucose and glutamine can be effectively targeted and restricted via diet-drug combinations, then every known major cancer is potentially manageable.


**Ben Stanger:**

Most cancers have a tendency to recruit many blood vessels via a process called angiogenesis. It is through this process that tumors are able to receive the oxygen and nutrients necessary for growth. However, some tumors, including pancreatic tumors, have a paradoxical feature: an "arid" microenvironment that's relatively deficient in oxygen and nutrients.

This suggests that there are likely to be certain pathways or mechanisms that cancer cells absolutely need in order to survive in a nutrient and oxygen-deprived microenvironment. If we can identify those dependencies, and target them, it may open the door to a new class of anti-cancer therapies.

**Saverio Gentile:**

It's been determined that when the potassium channel is stimulated, potassium exits the cell. Since potassium is a positively-charged ion, its exit from the cell results in an overall negative charge within the cell, and this negative intracellular charge becomes a driving force for calcium entry.[67]

When calcium enters, mitochondrial disruption is observed, which prevents the production of ATP (energy) and generates toxic chemicals such as "reactive oxygen species" (ROS). This means that the cell must find a way to make ATP, which it does through a process known as autophagy. Why is this important?

It's important because now we know that cancer cells need autophagy in order to survive. Further, we know that autophagy can be targeted by some drugs.[67]

One of the most important points of this approach is that the stimulation of potassium channels puts cells under stress. For example, ROS-dependent stress can be lethal, but cancer cells know very well how to counteract and compensate for this type of stress. In fact, this is likely why cancer cells survive so many other therapeutic approaches.

Through some of my research, now that we know some of the mechanisms that underlie the survival strategy of the cell, we can block them. More specifically, we can take a combinational approach by stimulating the potassium channel to drive the cancer cell into an energetic crisis (i.e., the need for ATP), and then blocking autophagy or we can eliminate the compensatory mechanism that cancer cells use to buffer ROS —ultimately killing the cancer cell.

**Susan Wadia-Ells:**

What's going into the gas tanks of breast cancer cells? As the metabolic theory of cancer shows us, killing a cancer cell means focusing on starving the cancer cell of its two major fuels: glucose and glutamine.[66] This is true for all types of breast cancer and for all types of cancer.

Triple-negative, and HER2-positive are two types of hormone-negative breast cancer. Unlike hormone positive breast cancer, these cancer cells often use more glutamine than glucose.

To put an end to any type of breast cancer, patients need to find health practitioners who will guide them in non-toxic ways that can block a tumor's access to glucose and glutamine.

**Adrienne C. Scheck:**

The ability of a tumor to grow well in a particular region will depend in part on the level of oxygen and food supply in that region. Tumor cells are glucose and glutamine-dependent, but the food a cell likes to use and the degree to which metabolism will function in a particular cell can differ, because at the genetic and epigenetic levels, there are countless differences. It's like rolling a boulder downhill—everything on its surface can change as it continues to roll.

**Manel Esteller:**

Tumors adapt to certain conditions by changing their epigenetic profile. About 90% of the genes in a metastatic tumor have the same epigenetic profile as the primary tumor; 10% differ epigenetically as a result of the adaptation that was necessary in order to escape the primary site and survive in the location of metastasis. Thus, these epigenetic changes may be critical for the survival of the metastatic tumor.[68]

# Today's predominant way of thinking about cancer

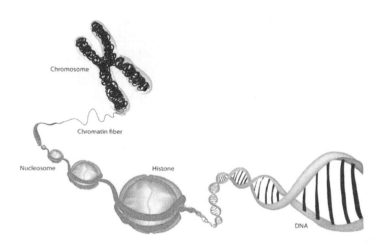

**Carlos Sonnenschein:**

The current dogma is over a century old, and was suggested by Theodor Boveri. Boveri speculated that cancer was caused by abnormal chromatin.[69]

Eventually, it was determined that DNA was the genetic material and that mutations in somatic cells cause cancer. However, with the advent of more sophisticated ways of exploring the problem, it's been discovered that those so-called driver mutations are present in normal cells.

In addition to our own experiments, it has been proven by others who have worked on the subject that the random somatic mutation theory is invalid.[70] Nonetheless, there are several sociological reasons that so many people keep harping on that dead horse.

**William Miller Jr.:**

The frame of reference for cancer research has been that cancers are stochastic, Darwinian, and selective. Cancer literature is all about selection of clonal lineages. I'm not saying selection doesn't matter—it does, of course. But what matters more is that cancer cells are self-referential and self-aware entities.[71]

When cancer cells agitate adjacent cells, they cheat by seizing resources that would not normally be available to a regular cell. This means that cancer cells are self-directed, selfish, self-referential agencies, and this is what permits coordinated action. In other words, this is what permits them to solve problems in cancer constituencies in competition with normal ecological players.

Attempts to suppress or extricate cancer along immunological lines is one way to approach the problem of cancer, but there is a big difference between thinking about cancer cells as self-referential and problem solving in their own right, and thinking about how to deploy T cells (i.e., use primary cells to combat cancer with immunotherapies and immune modulation). T cells are also self-referential problem solvers.[71]

All cells are smart and creative, and when they are viewed as such, different ways of approaching the problem of cancer can emerge. In essence, the takeaway is this: Cancer is much more than a matter of biochemistry.

**James DeGregori:**

I've been pretty vocal against the random mutation model. That said, I don't want to give off the impression that I don't think mutations are important.

I believe that environmental change drives evolution. An evolutionary biologist would certainly agree; cancer biologists, on the other hand, have been behind the eight ball in terms of understanding that the environment is a driver of cancer evolution.

To elaborate, what causes cancer to develop isn't just mutations; mutations occur all the time and we're absolutely loaded with them (including those that could be considered cancer-causing). However, the limiting factor for cancer development is a change in the tissue environment which favors mutant cells.[72]

For example, cigarette smoking indeed increases the frequency of mutations in the lungs, which contributes to a higher risk of developing lung cancer. But more importantly, it completely changes the environment within the lungs (we've all seen pictures of blackened lungs due to smoking) in such a way that it is rendered inconducive to normal lung cell types. In other words, it becomes an environment that is favorable for cells with cancer-causing mutations.

**Gábor Balázsi:**

The current paradigm for cancer is the random mutation-based initiation hypothesis, which is that a single cell initially develops mutations that may provide it with fitness advantages that allow it to grow faster or die slower, initiating tumor formation.

However, current knowledge shows us that there are alternative paths to cancer. For instance, a particular cell can undergo heritable, non-genetic changes.[33] This means that cells with unwanted properties can end up with a higher cell division rate and less death, which their daughter cells inherit—all non-genetically.

**Herbert Levine:**

For a long time, biologists have been looking at things from a relatively qualitative perspective, which is nonproblematic for many single-gene diseases; if a single gene is wrong or a single protein is nonfunctional, then the outcome is disease, and the proper way to treat it can be understood.

This paradigm hasn't really worked for cancer. Researchers have tried yet failed to identify individual genes that can enable things like cancer metastasis.[73] My perspective is that cancer and other complicated diseases are a combination of many different factors all working together in a very complex, yet organized way.

To address this type of problem, the use of mathematics and computational strategies are necessary. The focus should be on creating computational models that can predict how the various pieces are interacting,[74] as this will yield better progress on a shorter timeline than traditional biological approaches.

**Paul Davies:**

The standard somatic mutation theory posits that cancer is a product of genetic damage. I've never been convinced of that, because generally speaking, random damage to something is not going to improve its performance. It's like saying that taking a sledgehammer to the engine in my old Ford will suddenly turn it into a Ferrari.

If a cell finds itself in a poor tissue environment—for example, hypoxic (low oxygen), mechanically disrupted by wounding or subjected to altered electrochemical patterns - then the cell would think to itself, I've got a problem, but I remember the solution. And part of that solution is to revert to what it used to do, which is increase its rate of mutation.[75]

**Andriy Marusyk:**

The predominant way of thinking about cancers is that of the disease of genes, where accumulation of specific mutations causes progressively malignant behavior. The common assumption is that by studying these genes and pathways that they control will enable identification of "druggable" cancer-specific vulnerabilities, leading to better drugs and, hopefully, cures.

On a less reductionistic level, the picture is more complex. There is a good argument that tumor cells act as Darwinian units of selection (i.e., mutations modify chances of survival and proliferation, leading to outgrowth of fitter cells). On the other hand, there is strong evidence that a tumor cannot be fully understood without considering the role of differentiation programs, collective behaviors and interactions.[76]

In reality, there is a need to consider both Darwinian aspects (i.e., natural selection and adaptation) and differentiation programs; these are not mutually exclusive, but to date, there isn't a proper way to integrate them. This is just one challenge we need to address to understand the disease.

# CHAPTER 2: THE WHY

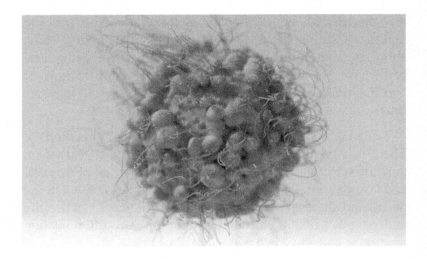

## Why are some types of cancer more aggressive than others?

**Yibin Kang:**

Two patients with stage 1 breast cancer come in for treatment. One patient will be successfully treated and the cancer will never metastasize or recur, while the other patient will undergo treatment, the cancer will develop resistance and metastasize, and the patient will die within a couple of years.

We know that some tumors are aggressive and result in very bad outcomes, while other tumors are less aggressive. But what dictates this? How can such different outcomes—despite the same type and stage of cancer—be explained?

The answer may lie in a category of genes called cancer fitness genes.

Most biologists tend to classify cancer-relevant genes as either oncogenes (which drive cancer growth) or tumor suppressor genes (which suppress tumor growth). This third category of cancer fitness genes cannot themselves cause cancer, but are essential for the cancer cell to survive and thrive under stressful conditions.[77]

This is important, because in order to progress from a primary tumor to metastasis, tumor cells must survive high levels of several types of stress, including hypoxic stress, metabolic stress (i.e., the need to access different kinds of nutrients), and mitotic stress (i.e., the need to replicate at high rates). These types of stress are not usually encountered by normal cells in a healthy person, which means cancer fitness genes are not important to the function of normal cells under normal conditions.[77]

Many cancer fitness genes become highly expressed as cancer progresses to a metastatic state, which indicates that they are driving cancer progression. One example of such genes cause cancer to downregulate their antigen presentation, which is crucial in order for the immune system to recognize a cancer cell as such and to attack it. Through suppression of the antigen-presenting system, cancer escapes immune surveillance, essentially becoming invisible to the immune system.[78]

Mouse model experiments have shown that targeting cancer fitness genes using small molecular compounds has therapeutic benefit. By using immunotherapies that not only keep the immune system active but also cancer fitness genes that suppress the immune system, we can essentially reactivate the host immune defense against cancer. Perhaps this is the pathway to a cure for cancer.


**Perry Marshall:**

This is the million-dollar question.

## Gábor Balázsi:

Both heterogeneity and plasticity will make a tumor more aggressive, but heterogeneity likely plays a larger role.[82]

This relates to evolutionary theory, because evolution and response to selection requires heterogeneity. To elaborate, cells diversify, and when they are under certain selection pressures, a subgroup of cells will do better than other subgroups. As a result, the process of fitness improvement continues.

## Robert Weinberg:

Multiple mutations will lead to an aggressively growing primary tumor. A byproduct of that aggressive growth will be the recruitment of normal host cells that are proinflammatory and reactive with the growth of the cancer cell.[83] Being so reactive, those cells will send signals that impinge on the cancer cells that recruited them. These signals will induce the cancer cell to acquire stemness (stem cell-like properties), invasiveness, and an ability to disseminate to distant sites.[83]

The initial steps of cancer formation do not necessarily require the formation of an entirely new colony; a cell with a single mutation can simply proliferate in situ where it arose. With the goodness of time, it may acquire additional mutations that allow it to progressively perturb the tissue around it, thereby converting that tissue into an environment that is increasingly hospitable to proliferation of the progeny of the initially mutated cell.

## Dominic D'Agostino:

A hallmark characteristic of cancers that are highly aggressive and metastatic is that there is a higher degree of mitochondrial damage.[79] There will be fewer mitochondria, which will be functionally different than the mitochondria in normal or benign cancer cells. Additionally, the mitochondria will have a greater proportion of immature as opposed to mature cardiolipin, which is a component of the inner mitochondrial membrane.[80]

These tumors have a very pronounced Warburg phenotype, meaning they ferment at very high rates of glycolysis (100-200 times more than normal).[81] In other words, aggressive cancers are very hungry for glucose and glutamine.

# Why and to where do cancers metastasize?

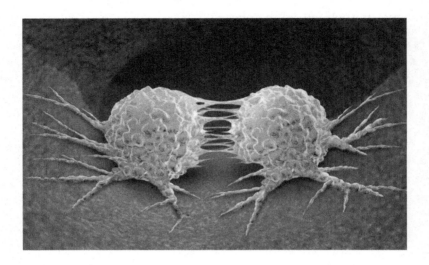

**Gábor Balázsi:**

This is a long-standing question. The well-known 'seed and soil' hypothesis, proposed by Stephen Paget in 1889, is based on the idea that not all seeds will grow well in all soils.[84]

This is a great idea, but how it works and what's behind it isn't well known. Why do certain tissue types develop metastasis more so than others, and what explains the fact that in many people, tumor cells will circulate in the body but not form metastases?

Likely, there is some type of lock-and-key mechanism at play between the target tissue and migrating cancer cell. The mutations and milieu of the original cell that leaves the primary tumor may enable features that fit a certain tissue type better than others, and this may relate to tissue types that have a common origin, embryonically.

Overall, it is not well understood why cancers tend to spread to certain areas of the body.

**Doru Paul:**

There are several explanations for metastatic cancer cells tropism, and the classical explanation is the mechanical one (i.e., capillaries in certain organs are fenestrated, meaning they have small holes that increase the flow of nutrients, oxygen, and other substances). This could explain why, in general, most frequent metastases occur in the lung and the liver where this type of capillaries are present.[85]

A recent breakthrough theory is that of Dr. David Lyden, who identified nanometric particles that are secreted by cancer cells and have on their surface a kind of protein GPS system, directing cancer cells toward certain metastatic locations (e.g., liver, brain).[86] This finding may help explain the old Paget's 'seed and soil' hypothesis.

**Robert Weinberg:**

It's been known for more than a century that cancers originating in one primary tumor site will tend to form metastases in specific, distant target sites in the body. The prevailing wisdom for a long time was that the cells preferentially migrate to certain sites in the body. For example, prostate cancer likes to form metastases in the bone marrow, while breast cancer likes to form metastases in the bone marrow and the lung.

The simple argument would be that these cancer cells actually have a tropism, which means that they are directed toward one organ or another. In other words, they tend to preferentially migrate to a certain organ.

The alternative point of view, which I embrace, is that when cancer cells start disseminating from a primary tumor, they're scattered everywhere throughout the body of a cancer patient; they are located in a great majority of sites, yet fail to succeed in launching a metastatic colony in most of those sites. But in some tissue sites, they do figure out a way to make a living with great facility.

My use of the term 'make a living' draws attention to the fact that when a cancer cell that's leaving the breast lands in the liver or the lungs, it's landing in a foreign tissue microenvironment where it is poorly adapted to thrive. The vast majority of cells that arrive in foreign territory will die as a result of the inability to adapt to the new biological environment.

When, on rare occasion, cancer cells figure out how to survive in the new environment, they will begin to create metastatic colonies that may ultimately undergo macroscopic growth. This can be readily observed in the clinic and can become life-threatening.

**Steve Gullans:**

Part of the answer simply has to do with blood supply, since it is in the bloodstream that primary tumor cells travel to other sites in the body, and some locations in the body are easier to access than others.

When a cell migrates into a tissue, it has to bind to the wall of the artery or the vein and migrate through it; this requires very specific mechanisms, similar to those used by circulating bone marrow stem cells that migrate to different tissues for repair purposes.

Think of the circulating cancer cell as having lost its attachment to the primary tumor but has a key on its surface that matches the lock in certain non-tumor tissues. This is something that is not completely understood, in part because it is such a dynamic system that changes very quickly.

**James Shapiro**:

The tropisms that cancer cells develop may be a reflection of the epigenetic changes that were triggered during the trauma or initial carcinogenic event. Just like different organisms occupy different ecological niches, different cancer cells may tend to go to different tissue niches in the body.

The body is a complex ecological system wherein the cells are under tight controls to stay where they are and do the things they're supposed to do; when they get out of control, we have to think of them as a new species with different behaviors and tropisms.

# Why might a benign nodule become malignant?

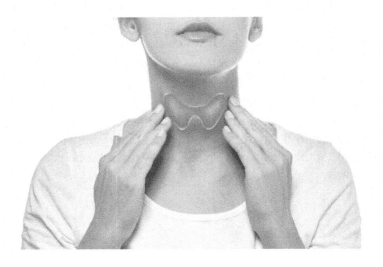

**Sui Huang:**

Do benign nodules have a tendency to become malignant? Is this something that people should be worried about?

The textbook view is that benign nodules can progress to malignant tumors, but it will depend on the tissue wherein they are located; in some cases, progression will be likely (obligate), and in other cases, progression to malignancy will almost never happen.

The newest finding is that in the tissues where small benign nodules become malignant, the malignant tumor is actually not a genetic descendant of the early benign nodule. This indicates that the entire tissue within which cancer arises may be sick in a way that facilitates the development of a malignant tumor.

In other words, cancer might not simply be the only result of a mutation turning one normal cell into a malignant cell, followed by proliferation of that malignant cell. An altered surrounding tissue likely plays a permissive role. This is both fascinating and puzzling.

**Mustafa Djamgoz:**

Early on in my research, one of my primary questions was this: Do cancer cells generate electrical signals? In hindsight, I realize that was a naive question, because every cell in the body generates electrical signals.

That question has since evolved to this: Is the difference between a benign cell and a malignant cell a matter of a difference in bioelectricity?

When cancer cells become aggressive, their membranes become electrically active.[87] It is as though these cells begin buzzing with electrical signals, a bit like neurons in an epileptic brain. It is this excitability which leads to aggressiveness and the ability to metastasize. At the core of this excitability is expression of embryonic voltage-gated sodium channels.

With all this in mind, I tell my students (jokingly) that before they begin their graduate studies, they should stick their finger into an electrical socket...just so they know the kind of force they're dealing with. This is how as a teenager I first experienced the impact of electricity on the body whilst building a radio transmitter.

**David Goode:**

When comparing low-grade or benign neoplasms to late-stage tumors, it becomes evident that the late-stage tumors have turned on more highly-conserved ancient genes than the early-stage tumors.[88] This suggests that as tumors progress, they shift more and more toward a unicellular life state and lose features of multicellularity, which may help them progress and adapt.

**Henry Heng:**

For a long time, it was assumed that a single cancer cell is very powerful, but we know now that an individual cancer cell is actually very weak on its own; there is growing evidence that heterogeneity is one of the most powerful strategies of cancer.[89]

With that in mind, I believe that whether a benign tumor becomes malignant has a lot to do with the genomic level of heterogeneity within the tumor, with karyotype changes driving the phase transition from benign to malignant. However, this is a topic that needs to be studied further.

# How cancer ultimately kills

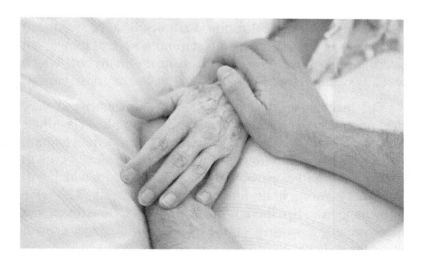

**Kenneth Pienta:**

A lot of people wonder how exactly cancer kills someone. The fascinating answer is that cancer in and of itself *doesn't* kill; it can take over[90] percent of a person's liver, for example, and that person can survive just fine.

However, when cancer grows in various places in the body, the body responds by releasing macrophages, cytokines, and chemokines that lead to things like cachexia (i.e., wasting syndrome) and ultimately death.[90] These growing cancers are referred to as swamp cancers, because in the process of trying to fight off the cancer, the patient's own body poisons itself; in essence, what's fatal is the swamp gas produced by the body as a result of the cancer.

**Yibin Kang:**

After I finished my postdoctoral research and started my independent research lab at Princeton, I focused primarily on the question of how cancer metastasizes, because that is ultimately why people die from cancer.

I came to the realization that death as a result of metastasis is like a final manifestation of several things that occur during the evolution of cancer—many of which actually occur before a person even knows they have cancer.

The mechanism of death by metastatic cancer can vary depending on the circumstances. For example, if a tumor metastasizes to the brain, there will only be a certain amount of room for the tumor to grow. As a result, continued growth of the tumor will cause compression of the brain, which will eventually disrupt brain function and cause death. The same thing happens when there is metastasis to the lung, liver, and other organs; it's organ failure as a result of cancer growth that causes death.

In other cases, the mechanism of death is more complicated. For example, metastasis to bone in the spinal cord can cause hypercalcemia, which can be life-threatening. Furthermore, since bone is the site of red and white blood cell production, metastasis to bone can lead to immune system disruption, which can leave the body vulnerable to stroke, blood clotting, and infection, all of which can cause death.

**Thomas Seyfried:**

The origination of the metastatic cell and ensuing metastasis is the process by which cancer kills most people. In order to control metastasis, it's critical to understand what metastasis is and what the cell needs in order to become metastatic, which is glutamine and glucose.[66]

**Sandy Borowsky:**

Immune reactions in cancer have been studied for a long time, but it wasn't until relatively recently that we've begun to exploit the fact that the host immune system—given the right stimuli—can eradicate cancer.

That said, we also know that the host immune reaction can be a double-edged sword, in that some patterns of inflammation are tumor-promoting, and therefore contribute to tumor growth. Likely, this is associated with the process of wound healing.[91]

With this understanding, it could be said that cancer creates a "wound," and the body's inflammatory reaction—designed to 'heal' it—actually promotes its growth, ultimately allowing it to be fatal.

**Brendon Coventry:**

Cancer is fatal when it grows in a haphazard fashion and begins to invade and damage organs. In most cases, disturbance to an underlying organ or function is what leads to the death of the patient.

In other cases, it's not entirely clear what makes cancer fatal, or why one person will succumb to cancer and another will survive it. Sometimes it has to do with the production of cachectin, which leads to cachexia or wasting of the patient. In this state, the patient can't harness any energy because the tumor is transforming normal tissue in a way that renders it unable to efficiently utilize energy.[90]

# If cancer kills, then why haven't cancer genes been eliminated through natural selection?

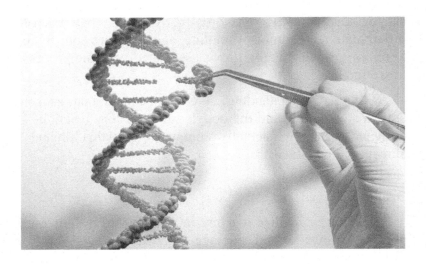

**Paul Davies:**

Why hasn't evolution eliminated cancer genes, if they kill us? The answer is that these cancer genes—whether involved in cancer promotion or suppression—have regular functions in healthy organisms, such as those related to the early stages of development and wound healing.92 We're stuck with cancer because cancer genes are foundational and cannot be eliminated.

In fact, it is sometimes said that a tumor is like embryonic development gone wrong; for example, during embryonic growth cells proliferate rapidly in a low-oxygen environment and move around a lot. These traits are also well-known hallmarks of cancer.

**Patrick Moore:**

The problem is that the genes involved in cancer development exist for a good reason: They fulfill important functions in normal cells. It's only when unfortunate circumstances and genetic accidents arise that cancer emerges. For example, the c-MYC gene codes for proteins that control the proliferation of certain cells that play a critical role in wound healing, embryonic growth, and immune system development.[93]

Under normal circumstances, this gene is turned on and off, whereas in cancer, it is persistently expressed (turned on). To prevent the proliferation of cancer cells, some have proposed the idea of cutting out the c-MYC gene using CRISPR technology. Doing so, however, can cause serious problems for the person, since this gene is very important for healthy cells and development.

**James DeGregori:**

If only cancers knew that their own aggressiveness would bring about their own end. One could draw an analogy between this and human activity on Earth: We are poisoning our own planet, yet not cognizant enough to do anything about it. The same could be said for tumors as they end up killing their own hosts, which is counterproductive.

# How do cancers behave "primitively"?

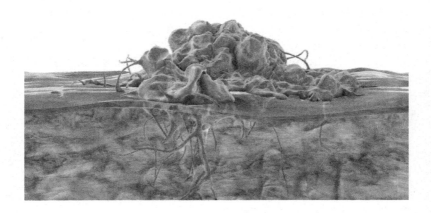

**Michael Levin:**

In our work last year, we showed that skin cells liberated from a frog embryo in a novel environment create a new creature, which we called a xenobot (i.e., a synthetic organism capable of organized movement).[95]

Watching this xenobot, one would never know that it has any relation to a frog, or that it was grown only from skin cells (no nerves). It has a totally wild-type frog genome with no changes whatsoever—no mutations and no oncogenes—yet it has rebooted its development into a completely novel form.

While there is a lot of research to be done here, I do think that tumors are a reboot of some kind of primitive multicellularity.

**Brendon Coventry:**

There's been a lot of work on the similarities between the role of the placenta and malignant invasive tumors,[16] which harkens back to the notion that there is some sort of ancestral behaviour going on with a tumor. In other words, tumors behave like very primitive things that are related to the very origins of mammalian placentation[248].

We know that bits of placenta (built of cells from both mother and fetus) can break off, travel throughout the body of a pregnant woman, become lodged in various areas, and be detected within the mother even decades later[94]; in essence, the mother has part of her child circulating in her body. This might seem like a scary thought, but it shows that the notion of metastasis is not exactly confined to cancer. We tend to reserve metastasis for tumors, when in fact, metastases occur in many non-cancerous situations. Sometimes 'benign' cells can break off from their tissues of origin, enter the lymphatics and lodge in lymph nodes, for example benign naevus cells occurring in lymph nodes or the blood circulation, or tissues from the placenta.[242, 243, 244, 245]

**David Goode:**

My hypothesis is that the transcriptomes of tumor cells change in such a way as to behave more primitively, which allows them to become more plastic, adaptable, and robust in order to better handle environmental stress.

In my lab, we look at signatures of loss of multicellularity using a model wherein tumor cells undergo a transition from a differentiated multicellular state to something that resembles a unicellular organism. This process can be studied by comparing the genes expressed in a human tumor to the genes of hundreds of other species, including those shared with very primitive, ancient single-celled organisms (e.g., bacteria, yeast), as well as the genes shared only with other mammals (which evolved much more recently).

We have found that tumor cells shut off the more recently-evolved genes and upregulate or increase their expression of very ancient genes that are conserved in bacteria and single-celled eukaryotes, as well early metazoan genes (i.e., genes that evolved early on in the process of multicellularity).[88]

# What is the atavistic theory of cancer?

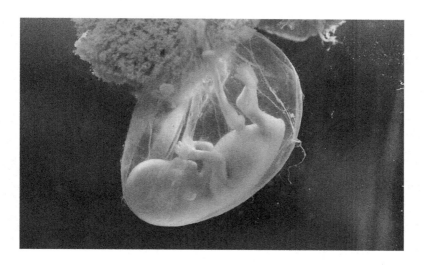

**Charley Lineweaver:**

The term applied to this concept is atavism, which is derived from the Latin *atavus*, meaning ancestor (it is sometimes called 'genetic throwback'). In essence, atavism is when features from earlier in a phylogeny or evolutionary history have not been successfully suppressed, and therefore appear in the adult form. In other words, those features do not disappear during early development.

For example, during the development of a human embryo, certain features that were present in the adult form of human ancestors are present, such as a tail and webbing between the fingers.[96] During embryogenesis, these features usually disappear; atavism is observed when these features do *not* disappear.

Other examples of atavism include adult horses with three toes (we know from the evolution of horses that they used to have five toes, then three, now one), and supernumerary (i.e., one or more extra) nipples in humans (we know that many of our ancestors have more than two nipples, including pigs, cows, and dogs). There are dozens of examples of morphological atavisms across many species.

The idea behind the atavistic theory of cancer is that in addition to morphological atavisms, there can be physiological atavisms.[97] For example, humans breathe oxygen, but oxygen has only been in the atmosphere for about 2.5 billion years. Prior to that, our ancestors were not using oxygen, which means they had cells that can operate in the absence of oxygen.

Human cells that have the ability to deal with an oxygen-free atmosphere are atavistic, and quite useful. For example, during intense exercise, an insufficient amount of oxygen reaches the muscles, and muscle cells change their metabolism to account for this (and produce lactic acid in the process).

The cellular ability to operate in the absence of oxygen is a holdover from 2.5 billion years ago, when cells had no option but to operate in the absence of oxygen.

When oxygen came along, a more efficient type of metabolism that can occur in the presence of oxygen developed, and this is what normal cells do under normal circumstances. Under other circumstances (such as overexertion of the muscles during exercise), cells revert to an earlier metabolic pathway that does not require oxygen.

Our atavistic model posits that cancer cells have reverted to doing things that our cells used to do a long time ago—namely survive in the absence of oxygen.[97] This ability has been stored inside ours cells because it is occasionally very useful to us.

**Kimberly Bussey:**

In my lab, we're looking at cancer from the perspective of atavism theory, which postulates that cancer initiation and progression represent reversions to ancestral unicellular phenotypes.[98] One of the things we're looking at is the role of stress-induced mutagenesis, and whether it can be detected in genome sequences of tumors.[99] Our goal is to determine the mechanisms behind it, and figure out the degree to which those mechanisms are conserved from the bacteria within which they were originally discovered.

Over the past 10 years, there has been a significant effort to catalogue the genes that are essential for development and reproduction. It is becoming apparent that the genes that are essential for multicellular organisms are not necessarily essential for unicellular organisms. However, when it comes to cancer cells, it is looking as though the reverse is true.

My lab is trying to determine which genes are essential for unicellular life versus multicellular life, and how we can use those networks to go after cancer.

**Paul Davies:**

Atavisms are well known to biologists, one of the most famous examples being supernumerary nipples (i.e. meaning one or more extra nipples). While most humans have two nipples, many of our ancestral mammalian species had more, and occasionally a modern human will as well. Our ancestors also had developmental pathways that led to the formation of tails. In humans, these pathways are normally suppressed, but if something goes wrong, they can still be expressed. These are examples of how modern organisms retain ancient latent abilities to deal with a problem.

In bacteria, certain genes are responsible for a very ancient response to stress, which is to deliberately increase their mutation rate.[99] For example, if bacteria are starving, they can elevate their mutation rate to look for other ways to metabolize.

Some colleagues of mine at Arizona State University found homologs of these genes in the human genome (older than about one billion years), which means that the same genes that allow bacteria to increase their mutation rate are retained in human cells, and allow them to increase their mutation rate in order to solve problems. This is what cancer does: It expresses these ancient genes and thereby elevates its own mutation rate.[98] This means that the high rate of mutation in cancer cells is not primarily due to a damaging environment (e.g., radiation) but is actually self-inflicted by the cancer cells in their search for a solution to a disrupted tissue environment.

# CHAPTER 3: THE HOW

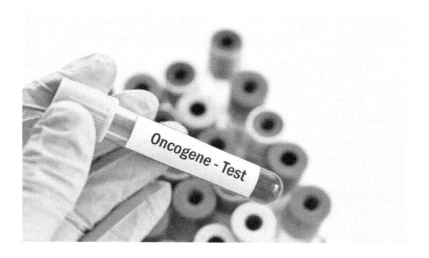

## How does cancer first start?

**Adrienne C. Scheck:**

There are some people who think that cancer first starts from a metabolic issue which causes genetic changes which lead to cancer. Personally, I would describe it differently:

Imagine that there are three balls of yarn in three different colors, labeled as genetic, epigenetic, and metabolic; cancer starts when those three balls of yarn are tossed into a room with a bunch of kittens who want to play; the result is a tangled mess, with each color being difficult to separate from the others.

I don't know if we'll ever be able to identify the very first thing that happens in a person who develops cancer.

In the lab, there are all kinds of ways to cause the formation of tumors, such as by transferring mutated genes or dysfunctional mitochondria into a healthy cell. But does what we do in the lab transfer to what happens in the human body?

**Michael Levin:**

One of the obvious ways that cancer starts is from broken hardware (e.g., sufficient mutation of genes and signaling proteins) resulting in abnormal cellular behavior.

What I find more interesting is when cancer begins even when there is nothing wrong with the hardware. In these cases, cells become electrically isolated from other cells, which can happen for various reasons.

As far as the electrically isolated cell is concerned, according to their bio-perception machinery, they are on their own, and therefore revert to behaviors designed to protect and further the goals of the self, which at that point, is just a single cell.

This process can be started by chemicals or oncogenes.[100] One of the first thing that happens after a strong oncogene is turned on is cells become electrically depolarized and disconnect electrically; they close the electrical synapses to their neighbors.

Using animal models, we have shown that it's possible to take perfectly wild-type animals and use an ion channel drug to temporarily block cells from having proper electrical connections to their neighbors. Under these conditions, the electrically isolated cells essentially convert to metastatic melanoma, even in the absence of carcinogenic exposure and mutation.[100]

**Thomas Seyfried:**

Otto Warburg clearly said that cancer starts from a chronic interruption of oxidative phosphorylation over time.[101] A perfectly healthy person is not going to wake up one day with a massive tumor; it is a gradual process.

We know that cancer starts when there has been damage to the oxidative phosphorylation system with a compensatory transition to fermentation. That transition to fermentation and the disruption of oxidative phosphorylation is what leads to genomic instability and somatic mutations that are seen in the nucleus of a cancer cell.[25] In other words, genetic damage and mutation are downstream epiphenomenon.

**James Shapiro:**

Around 1914, Theodor Boveri proposed that physical injury (e.g., scars on the body) can lead to the development of cancer,[69] even decades after the initial injury. Presumably, this is because physical injuries and scar formation disrupt normal cell division and growth.

In addition to physical injury, chemical injury, viral infections, and bacterial infections can lead to the formation of cancer. There are all kinds of processes that can disrupt the normal reproduction of cells and initiate a series of transformations that lead to cancer.

When it comes to identifying how cancer first starts, it is difficult to say, because we don't know a lot about the early stages of cancer. It's an area that people continue to research.

**Carlo Maley:**

To try to answer this question, I sometimes ask my students a similar question: When did cancer first start?

We tend to have a very human view of this because we are very concerned about cancer in humans, but it goes back to about two billion years ago, when all life on Earth was unicellular, like bacteria.

Consider for a moment that there's no way for a single-celled organism to develop cancer, because cancer is a problem of the cells of a multicellular body dividing out of control and then killing the host. Cancer only became a disease with the evolution of multicellular organisms, which occurred about two billion years ago in algae, and about 600 million years ago in animals.

I think of cancer as the hurdle that had to be cleared in order for life to evolve multicellular bodies, which require mechanisms for stopping uncontrolled cell division and for devoting cellular resources to the good of the body. Cancer seems to have disintegrated these mechanisms and evolved back into a single-celled form of life,[98] but since we don't have a record of that, it's hard to know how it happened. In any case, the critical change was the change from single-celled life to multicellular life.

# Can cancer start from a single cell?

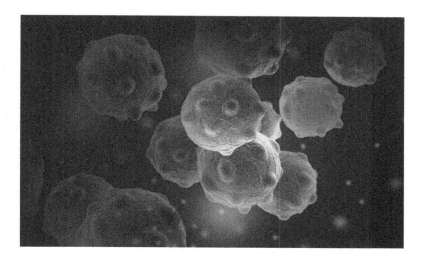

**Saverio Gentile:**

How could someone determine whether one cell—or which cell, for that matter—can generate a whole tumor? It's difficult to know, because it's still impossible to measure.

My view is that cancer starts from a series of insults on cells, and that it is highly improbable that a specific insult will affect only one cell; instead, it will affect a compartment of cells which will affect a body compartment (e.g., a patch of skin).

Humans are exposed to many pollutants and toxic agents which enter our body in a systemic way, which means that every single cell could potentially be in contact with any particular pollutant.

Then there is genetic. Change to the DNA is the basis of evolution but the outcome is not always helping an organism to survive. Sometime, gene mutation is the link to cancer as they can generate damaged proteins that, for example, are normally keep duplication under control.

**James DeGregori:**

The vast majority of cancers that arise in people are from a single event. Of course, there is incredible diversification after that event, but all of the cells in a tumor will share at least one truncal mutation (named as such because it is at the base of an evolutionary tree of cancer).[102] The event (e.g., a specific mutation or translocation) will be unique enough that the chance of it happening identically in multiple different cells leading to the tumor is very low.

Further, when that event happens in the cell, there will be a lot of what we call 'passenger' mutations already present in the cell. Since the mutations at the trunk will be present when the first event happens, we can be quite confident that an entire tumor arises from a single cell.

That said, people who develop one type of cancer are indeed more likely to develop a second, independent type of cancer.[103] This means there's something to be said about the presentation of an overall tissue or systemic environment that is conducive to cancer development.

**James Shapiro:**

Experiments carried out under very artificial conditions have shown that a single cell can grow into a tumor. Some people believe that cancers derive from a single cell, while others believe it is a disruption of the organization of tissues that makes a group of cells behave differently, and ultimately become cancerous.

Many tumors are heterogeneous, and when metastasis occurs, different clones of cells may be more prominent in certain areas of the body than others.[58] Variability is a biological property of cancer, and as cancers advance, they become more diverse and more complex in their genetic constitution.

**Gábor Balázsi:**

If we accept that cancer starts with a single cell that changes in genetic or epigenetic ways, then that cell has to divide and generate some sort of cell mass. What this process looks like will depend on the type of cancer, since some grow faster and/or require more oxygen and nutrients than others.

# How does cancer metastasize?

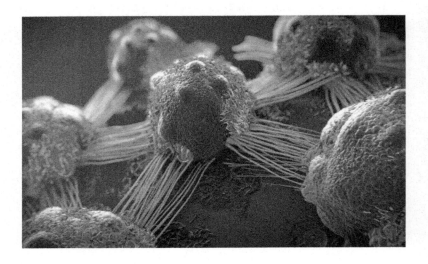

**Sandy Bevacqua:**

There are three major events that must occur for solid tumor cells to successfully spread throughout the body. First, they need to be able to attach themselves to the basement membranes that act as barriers in the body (every blood vessel, organ, and soft tissue structure in the body has a basement membrane around it).

Next, the cells need to produce enzymes to break a hole through the basement membrane and then motility factors to be able to wiggle their way through the basement membrane and into the bloodstream. Once the cells are in the bloodstream, some will get caught in a capillary bed somewhere in the body (e.g., liver, brain, lungs, etc.). Those cells then break open and wiggle through another hole they make in the membrane surrounding the capillary to make a tumor in the new location. This is how metastases occur.

In working with different individual tumors, I have noticed that some are very skilled at accomplishing these three tasks of metastasis, and others are not. In addition, some cancer cells have a genetically programmed preference for the organs they affect. These differences can now be used to target and effectively treat metastatic lesions.

**Adrienne C. Scheck:**

For a cell to metastasize, many different things have to happen: The cell has to break off from the primary tumor, enter the blood, lymph, or some other fluid within which to travel, exit the vessel that allowed it to travel, and then set up housekeeping in the new location.

Of the cells that end up being released into the blood (or other fluid) and traveling throughout the body, it's estimated that an astonishingly small number will actually form a metastatic tumor.

**Ana Soto:**

Every cell will proliferate unless it's inhibited by the tissue architecture. Cells in normal tissue are inhibited by the organization of that tissue.[104] For example, the first stage of an embryo is a zygote, which begins as a single cell that proliferates very quickly, but as soon as the cells begin to form tissues and organs, proliferation slows.

The rate of proliferation is controlled, among other things, by virtue of well-organized tissue. However, if the tissue is disturbed by something that alters communication among cells of different tissues, the cells will regain their ability to proliferate. Thus, they will proliferate like a tumor, travel, and metastasize.[104]

**Mustafa Djamgoz:**

It's a well-known fact that as a tumor grows, oxygen cannot diffuse sufficiently. This is a major trigger for things like angiogenesis, but it also turns on many genes and makes the cancer more aggressive.

Voltage-gated sodium channels normally open and close over a timescale of milliseconds (e.g., this occurs with each heartbeat, during muscle contractions, etc.), but under the hypoxic conditions of tumors, these channels stay open for thousands of milliseconds or seconds. This is a part of the cancer specificity of the sodium channel's function.[105] This causes a huge influx of sodium into cancer tissues, which can be visualized clinically using magnetic resonance imaging (MRI).

This influx of sodium leads to acidification of the cancer cells' surroundings, which leads to proteolysis (i.e., the breakdown or digestion of proteins and tissue matrix). As a result of this proteolysis, cancer cells are able to escape their physical barriers (e.g., basement membranes of organs) and enter their surroundings. In essence, this is how the motility and invasiveness of cancer occurs and once the cells hit upon a blood vessel and enter the circulation full-blown metastasis starts.[105]

**Kenneth Pienta:**

The bottom line is that no one actually understands the concept of a premetastatic niche as it applies to human beings.

We know that prostate cells express the CXCR4 receptor, which is normally found on white blood cells (i.e., cells that fight infection traffic to and from the bone marrow). When a white blood cell with CXCR4 is traveling through the bloodstream and needs to park, cytokines called stromal derived factor 1 (SDF-1) attract that receptor to park on an osteoblast (i.e., bone cell).[106]

It turns out that a prostate cancer cell does the same thing: As it is traveling through the bloodstream, it encounters a local SDF-1 gradient, and can actually knock off a white blood cell from its "parking spot." Then, the cancer cell sets up shop and stays dormant for some amount of time.[106]

As the cancer cell acclimates to the new environment, it starts to proliferate. While proliferating, it remodels its local environment and creates a niche construction that is favorable for it, such as by attracting new blood vessels and tumor-associated macrophages that help it grow and secrete enzymes that break down the local environment.[106]

In essence, cancer cells create their own little cancer swamp and continue growing. By the time a tumor is detectable via imaging, it's already composed of a billion cells (for reference, the tip of a thumbnail—about one cubic centimeter—represents about a billion cells).

# How do cancer cells communicate and interact with other cells in the body?

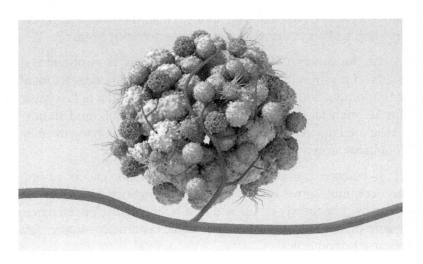

**Perry Marshall:**

What I've observed about evolution is that organisms of all types are extraordinarily cooperative. The traditional Darwinian narrative is about survival of the fittest, natural selection, competition, and differentiation. But the truth is that symbiotic relationships are all over the place—in our own backyards, and even between our mitochondria and chloroplasts.

I can only surmise that a tumor is a million Viet Cong soldiers and every one of them is a lone ranger, like Rambo, following their own agenda. And I can only surmise that they would find incredibly sophisticated ways to cooperate with one another, because that's how everything else in biology works.

Within the traditional Darwinian paradigm of survival of the fittest, natural selection, and the selfish gene theory (which is now completely obsolete), the only thing that would make sense is that everything on Earth would be like a tumor—

millions of Viet Cong soldiers with machetes, knives, and guns would be killing and eating everything in sight.

Is that what we see on Earth? No—we see things like coral reefs, and in a healthy human body, we seen an astonishing display of order and organization—the lungs, heart, muscles, nervous system—it's all marvelously cooperative.

**William Miller Jr.:**

What are the patterns of cellular activity that characterize cancer? Cancer cells follow the basic rules of cellular life in that they cooperate with one another, compete with one another, and actively trade resources and information among themselves and with adjacent cellular networks.[107]

Cancer cells cooperate with nearby normal tissues all the time. And since cells are cognitive, cancer growth and metastases are not random processes. Cancer cells make decisions, and they become different selves that do not have to abide by the same rules as other cells.

**David Goode:**

Cancer cells have some autonomy over their own growth and proliferation, and ignore normal anti-growth signals. Rather than listen to those signals, cancer cells come up with their own means of continuing to grow.

However, they are not entirely independent; there is a lot of evidence that tumor cells interact with and manipulate other cells in the microenvironment in such a way as to promote tumor cell growth.[108]

There are also different clones of cells within a tumor that will both compete and cooperate with one another. A lot of signaling occurs between cancer cells and the cells in their environment, as well as between different kinds of cancer cells within the same tumor.[109]

**Michael Levin:**

In a typical body where everything is working correctly and all the cells are electrically coupled into one coherent network, the self about which they are being "selfish" is rather large; since their electrical properties are smeared across tissues by gap junctions and electrical synapses, the cells cannot maintain an individual identity.[110] In some ways, they can't even tell where one cell's information structure ends and another begins.

But when those boundaries form and the cell becomes isolated from the giant network, it becomes very easy for the cell to determine the location of those boundaries. At that point, the cell continues being selfish about the needs of itself, at the level of that one cell.[110]

It has been shown that in some kinds of tumors, the tumor cells have lost communication with the healthy cells outside, but maintain good electrical communication internally. In other words, the tumor's internal communication network has become disconnected from the external communication network.[110]

Thus, it is the shrinkage and expansion of the boundaries of 'self' that occurs during embryonic development, during evolution, and during cancer that we need to track.

# Extracellular vesicle production in cancer

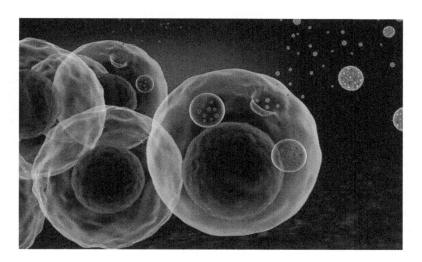

**James DeGregori:**

To quote biologist George Christopher Williams, "Evolution has no eyes for the future." In other words, a cell isn't able to say, "Hey, I should make premetastatic niches for my future offspring." Further, the cells that end up in the premetastatic niches may be very genetically unrelated to the cell that actually secreted the vesicles which helped form the premetastatic niches.

That said, the question must be asked: If one cell acquires the ability to make extracellular vesicles, how would doing so give that cell an advantage over the millions of other cells in the primary tumor? In the long run, it might favor the spread of the tumor itself, but the immediate question remains: What is the competitive advantage to the cell *at that moment*?

It's a question of immediate competitive benefit, and I think it must be the case that the ability to make extracellular vesicles provides a benefit that's manifested in the primary tumor, allowing the clone with that ability to expand to the point that it becomes more dominant within the primary tumor.

**Denis Noble:**

Cells release exosomes, which are very tiny packets of information about the regulatory state of the cells from which they came.[111] These exosomes are used as a form of communication between cells.

We also know that exosomes released by cancer cells contribute to a pathway that promotes metastasis,[112] allowing it to occur vastly quicker than it otherwise would. Although it's still controversial, there is some evidence that exosomes released by cancer cells prompt normal cells to become cancerous.[113]

**Carlo Maley:**

We know that cancer cells can bud off vesicles that can transport proteins and various hormones between cells.[112]

This relates to a phenomenon showing that after the removal of a primary tumor, many metastases can appear. This remained a mystery until it was discovered that—at least in some cases—the primary tumor releases antiangiogenic factors, which are hormones that suppress the growth of blood vessels.[114]

It follows that upon removal of the primary tumor (and therefore removal of antiangiogenic factors), metastases would be allowed to develop blood vessels and grow to detectable size.

The unanswered question becomes this: Why would primary tumors release antiangiogenic factors that suppress the growth of blood vessels?

**Gábor Balázsi:**

It is possible that cancerous cells are able to turn normal cells cancerous by releasing exosomes carrying molecular signals that promote this conversion.[113] That said, the tissue environment can stop a potentially cancerous cell; experiments have shown that a highly aggressive cancer cell embedded in a normal microenvironment can stop proliferating.[115]

I think that the exosomes and other signals definitely exist and go both ways, but how they ultimately play out is an interesting and unsolved question.

**Christos Chinopoulos:**

As of yet, we may not have a thorough understanding of the function and purpose of extracellular vesicles. This topic is being actively pursued with the purpose of cataloguing the contents of extracellular vesicles released by cancer cells.

Do their contents have the ability to coerce healthy tissues into becoming cancerous, or into sacrificing themselves for the needs of the cancer cells?

Investigating these types of questions, while potentially very valuable, has been technically challenging to accomplish due to the size of extracellular vesicles, and the difficulty in distinguishing them from cellular debris.[116]

# Primary tumor vs metastatic site communication

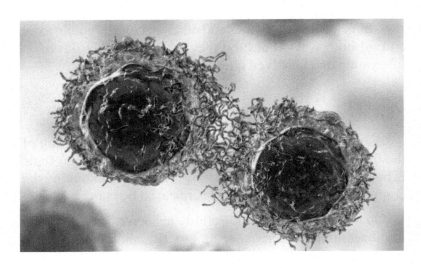

**Doru Paul:**

There are well-described cases showing that when a primary tumor is removed, regression or disappearance of metastases occurs.[117-118] However, the exact opposite phenomenon has also been shown (i.e., removal of a primary tumor was followed by the development of metastases).[114] It was determined that this is because a primary tumor can secrete angiostatin, which is a protein that inhibits cancer growth at a distance.

Another interesting concept is that metastasis can promote the development of the primary tumor. This ongoing interactions and communications between the primary tumor and metastases are very interesting. I think of it as a network that forms between the primary tumor and metastases, where the primary tumor might stimulate or inhibit the development of metastases, and the metastases might stimulate or inhibit the development of the primary tumor.

Of course, there could be the development of second metastases from the primary tumor and/or from the first metastases, so it's a very complex network.

**Steve Gullans:**

I am unaware of any coordination of action between a primary tumor and a metastasis. The mechanisms for metastasis are inherent in basic, normal functions of the body. For instance, bone marrow stem cells are released from the bone and travel to other parts of the body where they develop into other cell types.

**James DeGregori:**

There is evidence that the presence of a primary tumor can lead to metastatic niche remodeling, a process whereby the primary tumor may contribute to the development of a distant site that is favorable to metastasis (these sites are often called premetastatic).[119]

It's not clear why that happens, because we have to keep in mind that a tumor doesn't have agency. In other words, the tumor is not thinking, *I'd like to create a nice spot in the liver for my children*. Instead, it's more like there is something about the primary tumor that is creating a systemic change that makes it more likely for metastasis to seed in distant organs.

**Seyedtaghi Takyar:**

I would say that a primary tumor is probably not driving or steering the metastatic site, because we often find metastatic sites without the existence of the primary site.[120] In other words, metastasis will be identified, but we will be unable to find a primary tumor. In these cases, it's likely that the primary tumor died and no longer exists, while the metastatic site lived on.

**James Shapiro:**

The ways in which a primary tumor will affect metastasis or vice versa run the gamut, from primary tumor cells being in continued contact with metastasis, to metastatic cells being completely independent and having no communication with the primary tumor.

# Evading the host's immune defenses

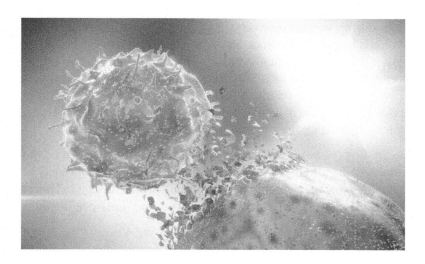

**Christos Chinopoulos:**

One trick that tumor cells have in their pocket is that they can become immunologically blank, meaning that they do not show evidence of being foreign in the tissue where they are located.[121] This means that a cancer cell that is in the liver, for example, will appear to the host's immune system (i.e., the immune cells that constantly circulate and surveil the body for foreign particles) as part of the normal liver tissue.

**Samantha Bucktrout:**

Cancers are amazingly adaptable and plastic, and there's a constant battle between the immune system and a particular type of cancer. One way cancer evades the host's immune system is by downregulating major histocompatibility complex (MHC) molecules, which the immune system uses to see any cell in the body.[121]

**Kenneth Pienta:**

Macrophages are white blood cells that the immune system uses during wound recovery (e.g., getting rid of bacteria in the wound, helping with scar formation). By constantly breaking down the environment around a tumor, cancer has the ability to fool these macrophages into thinking that a cancerous tumor is a wound.[122] As a result, macrophages (referred to as tumor-associated macrophages) go to the site of the tumor and try to "clean it up" like they would a wound.

In the process, however, these macrophages actually feed the cancer cells, and thereby promote cancer growth. It is a vicious cycle that allows cancer cells to continue proliferating.[122] This is why cancer is often referred to as the "wound that never heals."

When it comes to prostate cancer, we know that up to 50% of the tumor mass is actually composed of these tumor-associated macrophages.[123]

**Jo Bhakdi:**

Normal cells in the body have certain mechanisms for signaling to the immune system that something is wrong with them. For example, if a cell is infected with a virus, it will tend to display evidence of that virus on its surface.[124]

It is as though cells have a reporting system for alerting the immune system to the presence of an alien or mutated protein by way of showing on its surface what is inside of it. The immune cells respond to that reporting system, and will usually kill the compromised cell.

This reporting system or mechanism involves a number of proteins. If this mechanism is stopped or becomes nonfunctional, then the immune system will have no way of knowing which cells are infected by a mutated protein, virus, or is otherwise compromised. In essence, compromised cells become invisible to the immune system.

While not fully understood, cancer cells have a way of disrupting the reporting system so that the cancer cells do not display anything on their surface alerting the immune system to a problem. This is just one example of how cancer cells can hide from the host's immune system.

**Carlo Maley:**

The immune system often recognizes cancer (and other) cells by the presence of abnormal or mutant proteins on their surface, which makes the cells appear foreign to the immune system.

Once cancer cells develop enough mutations, the immune system will recognize the resultant abnormal proteins. However, cancer cells can evade the immune system by not expressing those mutant proteins, thereby silencing the system that alerts the immune system to the presence of them.[121]

Cancer cells also send out hormones to recruit regulatory T cells that are part of the normal ramping down of the immune response.[125] In essence, this tells the immune system "There's nothing to see here, move along."

In some cases, cancer cells will express cell surface signals that tell immune cells to stop reacting to them, and to in fact kill other immune cells.[126]

Some of the methods cancer cells use to evade the host's immune system require cooperation (e.g., more than one cell to produce a hormone to attract regulatory T cells), but some of them can be done by a single cell (e.g., suppressing the antigen detected by the immune system, killing off immune cells, etc.).

**Brendon Coventry:**

Alistair Cochran led a research group at UCLA that showed that the lymphocytes that are closer to a tumor are less responsive than the lymphocytes that are further away from a tumor.[127] In other words, the further from the tumor, the greater the responsiveness and the lower the degree of inhibition of lymphocytes.

It was postulated that this gradation was caused by the release of certain chemicals by the tumor. Through further research in my own lab, we found that tumors indeed produce factors which downregulate immune cells that are close to a tumor[246]. Based on these findings, Steven Rosenberg's group and others have shown that renewing lymphocytes will lead to a greater response against a tumor than activating lymphocytes that are switched off inside a tumor.[128]

# Do cancers evolve their own immune system?

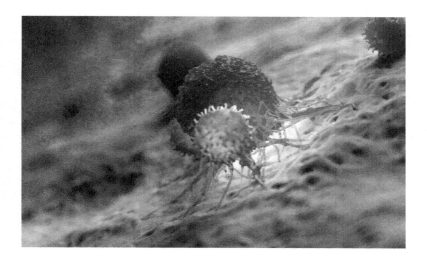

**Brendon Coventry:**

The tumor is a remarkable entity that has its own immune system locally and affects the systemic immune system. We've come to discover that they're not necessarily the same thing; what's happening locally in the tumor deposit is not necessarily what's happening systemically in the periphery (e.g., the blood).

What we end up with is a fascinating situation where this entity is growing inside the body, and will either remain local or spread throughout the body. When it spreads, it almost takes on a different persona and develops its own way of affecting (or not affecting; tolerating) the host's immune system both locally at the site of each tumour deposit and systemically.[247, 248]

**Gábor Balázsi:**

When tumors first begin to form, I don't think they have their own immune system in any way. As they develop, they will sometimes be attacked by the host's immune system, at which point it will become an evolutionary survival game—with selection for the cancer cell to figure out a way to trick the host's immune system.

The cancer cell can not only avoid being attacked, but can also use host immune cells as sources of protection and growth. Cancer cells that are able to do this will grow faster, become heterogeneous faster, and evolve an immune system in the sense that more and more immune cells (e.g., macrophages) will become tumor-friendly and may actually fuel cancer growth.[125,129]

**Perry Marshall:**

Tumors develop semi-autonomous behaviors that are entirely different from the host's. They recruit blood vessels, food, nutrients, and oxygen. They bamboozle the host's immune system and send signals that say, "Everything's okay over here, don't worry about us." Looking at biology through a symbiotic lens, it would only make sense that cancer cells collectively form entire defense systems and ecosystems against the host until the host is dead.

# How does cancer remission occur?

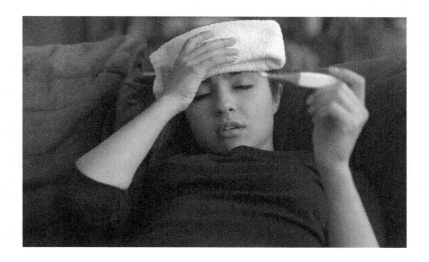

**Ronald Brown:**

It's been shown that fevers are associated with remission of tumors.[130] I think this has to do with the fact that most people who have a fever will lose their appetite, and will therefore eat less. If there is less phosphorus going into the body as a result of eating less, then the body will have a chance to "clean up" and excrete sequestered phosphorus (see my answer to question #3).

**Perry Marshall**:

How is it that cancer cells get off track and forget who they are? How could they be convinced to go back to being regular tissues? Michael Levin has demonstrated how—he's been able to make tadpole tissue become cancerous using bioelectric fields, and then 'normalized' that same tissue (i.e., gotten it to become non-cancerous again).[100]

We all know that some people have spontaneous remission, where the cancer suddenly disappears and no one knows how. There must be a mechanism by which cancer cells have an epiphany and remember who they are.

**Michael Levin:**

There are data suggesting that embryonic environments can normalize cancer.[131] Work in mice, chicken, and in regenerating amphibian limbs has shown that cancer cells put into an actively patterning environment (i.e., an environment where cells are getting very strong cues about what they should be doing) get normalized and participate as part of the correct morphogenesis.

A very straightforward and effective procedure is to artificially enforce the correct voltage map with the use of ion channel drugs or optogenetics (e.g., by introducing novel light-gated ion channels), resulting not only in the normalization of existing tumors, but prevention of tumor development.[132]

**Ana Soto:**

How is it that a large number of children with neuroblastoma cure spontaneously?[133] Many experiments have been done to explore the question of how cells that once belonged to a cancer can be normalized, and it's been demonstrated that normal tissues can induce cancer cells to behave normally.[134-136]

To elaborate, the relationships between different cell types can be affected by a carcinogen to the point that communication between them is weakened. When communication is weakened, cells that have the propensity to proliferate very fast are no longer inhibited in forming complex structures, and as a result, they begin proliferating and moving.

However, when these cells are put back into a normal environment with normal cells, the normal cells not only inhibit that proliferation, but induce normal behavior and the expression of normal proteins.

Importantly, Gil Smith from the National Cancer Institute demonstrated that there must be the right ratio of normal cells to cancer cells in order for normalization to occur, which is 10:1, and in some cases just 5:1. This indicates that the normal cells have to make junctions with the cancer cells in order to form structures and induce normalization.

**Gary Foresman:**

Patients of mine who have had radical remission from cancer made shifts on all levels because they realized that healing comes from something more than just a diet change, or just an exercise change, or just starting a meditation program—it's really about doing all of these things.

I think that most people cannot heal from certain ailments by putting all of their eggs in one basket (i.e., focusing on just one thing, like just exercise or just diet). But for something as serious as cancer, patients need to implement change on all levels of their lives.

I tell my patients that healing from cancer is a full-time job. To build a foundation of health, I tell people to set aside an hour a day for healthy exercise, an hour a day for meditation, and an hour a day for healthy eating and food preparation.

Far too many doctors tell their patients what to remove from their lives in order to heal (e.g., junk food, hours of TV every day) without addressing the things they need to add to their lives. It's important for patients to shift their awareness to the things that are fulfilling to them, and to add things to their lives that bring them joy (perhaps a sense of joy similar to the one felt while engaging in unhealthy habits).

# SECTION 2

# APPROACHES TO UNDERSTANDING, DETECTING, AND TREATING CANCER

# CHAPTER 4: UNDERSTANDING CANCER THROUGH RESEARCH

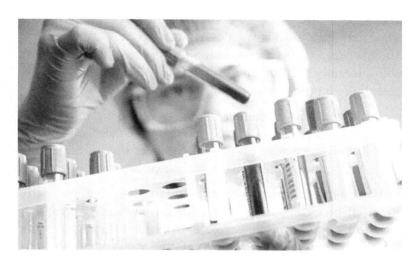

## What's missing in our understanding of cancer?

**William Miller Jr.:**

What does the microbiome of a particular type of tumor look like? What does the metabolome look like? What about the resource training? And how does one type of cancer, such as colon cancer, differ in these ways from other types of cancer? Scientists have accomplished remarkable things in cancer treatment and made terrific progress, but every single one of these questions remains unanswered.

We are beginning to understand that certain bacterial strains in colonic microbiomes are associated with a higher incidence of cancer. We know that patients with inflammatory bowel disease (IBD) (i.e., ulcerative colitis and Crohn's disease) have a much higher incidence of cancer because they have a breakdown of the normal gut barrier integrity.[137]

This breakdown must mean that there are cross-transfers of microbial life from the colon into the gut lining which is abnormal and somehow contributes to tumorigenesis.[137] Since we don't know how to stop this process, many patients with ulcerative colitis end up getting colectomies, which is essentially a colon amputation.

When it comes to cancer treatment, there are many open questions which, if answered, could lend themselves to a new and efficient way of attacking cancer that goes beyond the recruitment of additional immune cells.

For instance, current cancer treatments are primarily aimed at blocking the proliferation of clonal lineages, and essentially lining up cancer cells in order to try to execute them. But what would happen if the focus were to shift toward blocking the *senome* of cancer cells?

Similarly, perhaps the senome of the normal cell can be made more acute, or improvements can be made to the way cancer cells co-partner with nearby cells. In order to accomplish this, we'd have to understand how organisms gain information from the environment, intelligently assess it, and measure it—critical components which are missing from our understanding of cancer.

**Brendon Coventry:**

There is a lot we still don't know about cancer, especially when it comes to treating it. For example, are smaller or larger doses of treatment better? Should treatment be delivered more (or less) frequently or in intervals? Is there a rhythm in the immune system function in cancer patients which might determine the effectiveness of treatments depending on the timing of administration; or even make treatment less effective or make tumors grow faster?[249,250,252] Is there a route of drug delivery that is superior to others (e.g., subcutaneously or intradermally vs. intravenously)? Should a tumor be resected right away, or is it more beneficial to deliver immunotherapy first?

The answers to these important questions perhaps surprisingly remain largely unknown.

I think we really need to urgently go back over and look at much of our past experience and collective knowledge to 're-group' to make sure we are truly fully comprehending what we have been learning; and that we are not missing the essential cross-linking of vital information that can help our mission[247, 248]. I suspect we may not be fully utilising many of the answers we now already have in front of us within the literature.

**Carlo Maley:**

One of our blind spots in cancer biology has to do with the dynamics of what are called micrometastases, which are too small to show up on MRI, PET, or CT scans. Micrometastases are essentially invisible to us, and as a result, it's hard to know how common they are.

Some researchers have identified single epithelial cells in bone marrow (which shouldn't be there), but they do not tend to grow.[138] Micrometastases, on the other hand, can sometimes blow up into detectable and deadly masses.[139]

**Manel Esteller:**

First, we need to develop a complete profile of all the epigenetic changes that are going on in cancer cells, as well as the cells involved in other disorders. Second, we need to use that knowledge to identify biomarkers that will predict the outcome of the disease or help in the selection of better therapies.

**Robert Gatenby:**

There are several reasons the dominant theory of carcinogenesis does not fit well with evolutionary theory, nor with some empirical observations. In general, we've tended to be cell-centric in that we view the cancer cell as isolated in itself, as opposed to part of a system of tissues and normal cells. We are also gene-centric that the evolution of cancer is entirely related to genetic mutations. In evolution, the genome is simply the "mechanism of inheritance." Evolution occurs through the interactions of environmental selection forces and the phenotypic properties of the cell. The genome is more like a record of these events than their direct cause.

When it comes to cancer treatment, there is this idea that the more cancer cells that are killed the better. Rather than focus on killing as many cancer cells as possible, which will also lead to the death of normal cells, it's necessary to understand how to kill cancer cells selectively, without harming normal cells.

**George Calin:**

In most diseases, including cancer, clinicians do not have a clear understanding of why the same type and stage of disease that presents in two patients who are of the same age, gender, and race will behave very differently.

# Insights from tumor organoid models

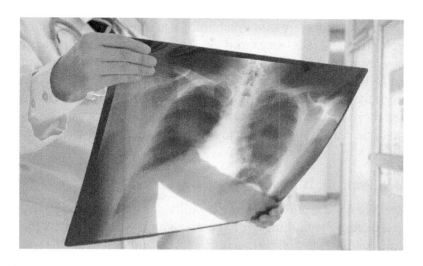

**Robert Weinberg:**

Traditional methods for studying cell propagation in the lab involve forcing cells to attach to the bottom surface of a Petri dish and observing how they proliferate and behave thereafter. However, since this is proliferation in 2D, it misrepresents the reality of what goes on in living tissue, which is a 3D world.

Organoids represent a mechanism or technology for propagating cells in a 3D matrix rather than on the bottom of a Petri dish. By putting cells into a particular type of gel with the right mixture of growth-stimulating factors, the cells exhibit many of the attributes associated with the cells in living tumors.

**Doru Paul:**

My colleagues at Weill Cornell are working on the creation of organoids for the study of pancreatic cancer. In essence, a tumour organoid is a 3D- construct that mimics, as accurately as possible, the type of growth that would occur in its corresponding in vivo organ.

While tumor organoid technology is superior to the use of Petri dishes, the organoid is still an entirely artificial environment, in large part because of the absence of immune cells. Researchers are trying to develop organoids that include immune cells, but there is still a lack of cellular variety (there are more than 30 different immune cells in the body). This is just one reason organoid research is still in its infancy.

**Benjamin D. Hopkins:**

When we receive a tumor to study at my lab, we begin by dissociating it into individual cells, which we then use as the cellular basis for creating tumor organoids. The goal is to recapitulate the tumor microenvironment as best as possible, within reason.

We provide custom media components to different tumor types in an attempt to make them look as similar as possible to the tumor from which they came. Through this process, we may end up with hundreds or thousands of copies of the same tumor.

Next, we run dose-response experiments, through which we deliver every drug that the patient could theoretically receive. This allows us to assess the sensitivity of the tumor to each drug, and compare the relative drug sensitivities of each tumor to every other tumor we've tested.

In doing so, we can say that a given tumor is more or less sensitive to a particular therapy, and we can compare that to the drug that the patient would normally receive in the clinic. For example, patients with ovarian cancer receive cisplatin (a platinum-based chemotherapy) in cycles until they no longer respond. We can use the relative sensitivity data from our models to identify drugs that may be more effective.

The most interesting part of all of this is that, while tumors were originally classified by the tissues from which they arose (e.g., breast cancer arises from the breast, liver cancer arises from the liver, etc.) and not necessarily by molecular characterization, a particular tumor type or set of tumors arising from *different* tissues often have shared, specific genetic mutations which give rise to a specific drug sensitivity.

The organoid modeling approach allows us to correlate genetics to therapeutic response, and identify very specific patterns of combination sensitivities. For example, in a KRAS-mutant tumor there can be sensitivity to an MEK inhibitor, which gives rise to secondary sensitivity to another drug that would not usually be very toxic to a normal cell.

This means that tumor cell-specific vulnerabilities can be created by leveraging the effects of one drug in order to sensitize a tumor to a second drug. These vulnerabilities tend to fall into set metabolic patterns and predispositions, whether they are being driven by the location or genetics of the tumor.

**Jyotsna Batra:**

It's rather difficult and time-consuming to establish organoids from every patient. That said, it is much easier for some tumors than others.

The beauty of using organoids is that the outcomes yielded come from the heterogenous groups of cells within tumors, which means organoids from different patients will not necessarily deliver the same outcome. This type of research provides a terrific opportunity to take into account the importance and impact of the heterogeneity of cancer.

# Current cancer research projects

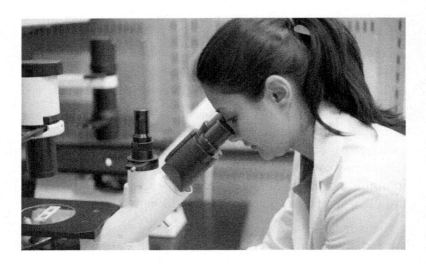

**Jake Becraft:**

Over the past 20 years, the Human Genome Project has resulted in a wealth of data, especially in terms of the biomarkers that exist inside or outside of a cell in a given disease state. This has led to more and more attempts to improve therapeutic specificity, meaning the ability to target specific cells in order to improve treatment outcomes. Most people have approached this issue of specificity by targeting surface biomarkers in order to deliver messenger RNA (mRNA) into the correct cells.

At Strand, we're taking a different approach—one that does not require us to focus on the selectivity of RNA uptake.140 This is because we have programmed mRNA to activate and actuate its therapeutic payload only once it's reached its final destination (targeted recipient cell).

To accomplish this, we have encoded genetic sensors on the sequence of the mRNA itself. The biological circuitry will process the output of these sensors at the genetic level, and turn on or off whichever genes are encoded on the vectors.[140] In other words, the therapeutic itself will be able to make a decision based on logic through 'AND' and 'OR' gates, similar to the way in which early computers utilized the decision-making process. Only now, the decision will be about whether to express the therapeutic output that's been encoded on the vector itself.

Since the mRNA molecules are equipped with this logical decision-making capability, the lipid nanoparticles (a cutting-edge delivery method)[140] carrying them only need to reach the right tissue. In other words, there can be heterogeneity in the types of cells to which the therapeutic is delivered, as long as a significant portion reaches the target tissue.

I like to think about it like this: The lipid nanoparticle will bring the mRNA to the right neighborhood, and the mRNA will make sure it gets itself to the correct house.

There are all sorts of creative bioengineering solutions for improving the therapeutic potential of mRNA molecules; it's just a matter of intense bioengineering.

We will be conducting our first human clinical trial in 2023, which will be in the solid tumor immuno-oncology space. For the foreseeable future, we will be scaling out the capabilities of our platform, building improved breakthrough drugs, and continuing to attack new disease areas using this technology, all in the quest to bring mRNA therapies forward to treat and cure more disease and increase human wellness!

**Samuel Sidi:**

In 1996, I discovered the zebrafish model by accident, and I've never stopped using it since. I quickly recognized the power of this model, which rests upon the distinction between the reverse genetic and the forward (unbiased) approach to drug and genetic screening.

The reverse genetic approach is inherently biased in the sense that the researcher must begin with a gene of interest and a hypothesis about that gene. Phenotypic analysis is done following disruption of the gene of interest.[141]

In contrast, the unbiased approach *begins* with a phenotype and the right biological question; it does not require a hypothesis or even a preconception of the answer to the question.[141] For example, researchers who were interested in the development of wings in flies (but had no hypothesis or genetic knowledge pertaining to this interest) used the unbiased approach by *randomly* mutating the genome of the fly and examining thousands of progeny for the phenotype of interest (i.e., improperly developed wings). At that point, identifying the gene that produces that phenotype is only a matter of performing whole-exome sequencing on the mutant fly.

Historically, this approach has been limited to invertebrate models (e.g., flies, worms) for reasons of feasibility; using mice, for example, would require a ton of space and money, since thousands of mice would be needed. As a result, the use of this unbiased approach in investigating questions relevant to vertebrates—and more specifically human disease and development—has been limited.

This is where the zebrafish model has become invaluable: Not only is the zebrafish a vertebrate and therefore more genetically and pathophysiologically similar to the human, but it's small, so many more can be grown in a small facility.[142] And crucially, the researcher is never limited by the number of embryos, because every female can produce up to 300 embryos per week.

Many people in the zebrafish field apply the unbiased approach, typically to identify genes involved in development, cardiac function and regeneration, stem cell function and replenishment, and human hematological and behavioral phenotypes.

I am a bit unusual in that I'm applying this approach to drug discovery in cancer. By using the zebrafish model, we can overcome a major obstacle in this field, which is to find drugs that are not only efficacious, but *nontoxic* to the animal as a whole.[143]

Screening for drugs that restore sensitivity to radiation in cancer cells grown in a Petri dish will identify drugs that are effective, but will leave out the most important information, which is whether the drug is toxic.

The issue has always been about killing only—or at least preferentially—the tumor cells, and leaving the healthy cells unharmed.

Using the unbiased approach in zebrafish, we have found something completely unexpected: A kinase enzyme called IRAK1 is absolutely crucial to the ability of the zebrafish to survive ionizing radiation.[144]

In collaboration with many researchers, we have confirmed that this is indeed a tractable and actionable target for restoring cancer cell sensitivity to radiation in human patients. We are currently working on the development of a nontoxic drug that targets this enzyme in order to overcome resistance to radiation therapy in very specific solid tumor types.

By asking the right question at the right time with the right assay and the right team of people, it is not unreasonable to think that progress in this direction will occur rapidly, within a matter of years as opposed to decades.

This strategy of unbiased screening is leading to real potential and progress in the treatment of cancers that would otherwise be incurable.

**Manel Esteller:**

I study something that's pretty new in the field of oncology called transdifferentiation, which is when one tumor type becomes another tumor type by completely changing its epigenetic setting in response to a chemotherapeutic drug (i.e., in an attempt to escape the effects of the drug and survive). For example, acute lymphoblastic leukemia (ALL) can become acute myelogenous leukemia (AML),[145] and prostate adenocarcinoma can become neuroendocrine prostate cancer.[146]

In the coming years, I believe the use of single-cell technologies to study bulk samples will provide a lot of answers in the epigenetic field, and that big data analysis tools will be employed to analyze DNA methylation in the context of multiomics. Hopefully, this research will lead to the development of more specific epigenetic therapies.

**Sendurai A. Mani:**

Despite the advent of advanced diagnosis and treatment options, metastasis accounts for more than 90 percent of deaths among cancer patients. Unfortunately, there are no treatments available for patients with metastasis. The ultimate goal of our research is to target and successfully treat metastasis. To accomplish this, we need to understand the biology behind it.

We and others have demonstrated that the carcinoma cells, which are initially confined to the primary tumor site by the continued expression of cell-cell adhesion molecules, acquire mesenchymal morphology, increased migration, invasion, and metastatic properties by activating a latent embryonic program, known as epithelial-mesenchymal transition (EMT).

In addition, during metastasis, cancer cells leaving the primary site recreate tumors histopathologically similar to their tissue of origin at the metastatic site. Therefore, we hypothesized and demonstrated that the cancer cells also acquire stem cell properties via EMT in addition to migratory and invasive capacities. Because both cancer stem cells (CSCs) and the EMT program are independently shown to be responsible for promoting metastasis and the acquisition of resistance to standard of care therapies and we have found that these two are indeed intertwined, we put forward the notion that the EMT-signaling pathways may offer a diagnostic and therapeutic window for detecting and treating metastasis. At present, our laboratory is investigating the biology of metastasis at the molecular level and developing ways to diagnose and treat metastasis.

Specifically, we are studying how an incomplete transition, whereby cells gain mesenchymal and stem cell properties without losing epithelial properties, may promote metastasis. We have termed this 'hybrid EMT.'[147]

We also use single-cell RNA sequencing to study the interaction between cancer cells and immune cells. By sequencing primary tumors and metastases, we can study cancer cell signals versus immune cell signals and hopefully reveal ways to intervene in those signals. Additionally, we're exploring spatial transcriptomics, which allows us to investigate the type of signaling that occurs between tumor cells and the microenvironment.

Lastly, we are using multiplex immunofluorescence, whereby we can stain up to 40 markers in a single tumor and characterize various cell types within that tumor.[148] This technology is helping us to understand the spatial orientation of tumor cells and immune cells.

**Kenneth Pienta:**

We are taking three different approaches to the study of cancer:
1. We're actively testing how we can stop macrophages from getting into the tumor microenvironment at all, and how to turn them off if they are already there. Understanding this would be a major step forward in controlling cancer and the production of swamp gas, which is ultimately fatal (see my answer to question #13).
2. In addition to looking for therapies that might kill cancer cells, we are trying to identify therapies that will inhibit the poisons that cause wasting syndrome. In other words, we are looking for ways to treat wasting syndrome as a result of cancer as opposed to the cancer itself.
3. Based on the belief that poly-aneuploid cancer cells are central to the growth of tumors within the tumor microenvironment, we're developing strategies to directly target them (see my answer to question #27a).

**Maria Casanova-Acebes:**

The focus of my postdoctoral research was on embryonic macrophages, which are part of the innate immune system. At two months of human gestation, embryonic macrophages are present (in the absence of T and B immune cells) and operate not only during disease, but also during homeostasis.[149]

For example, a population of macrophages in the brain called microglia are necessary in order for synapses to form proper networks of connection. If a person does not have microglia, they will have problems with cognition and motor function, so these macrophages are necessary for development.[149]

During organ development, morphogenesis and cellular turnover is necessary for growth. This is because there is a certain number of cells that the tissue in any given organ can hold, which is established by the proliferation and elimination of cells.

One hypothesis is that in non-small cell lung cancer, the tumor cells somehow mimic or recapitulate the program of morphogenesis by embryonic macrophages, and that in this way, embryonic macrophages may promote metastasis.[150]

Moving forward, the goal is to better understand whether embryonic macrophages demonstrate prometastatic potential in other organs as well, as this would bring us closer to being able to systemically target this population of macrophages in several types of cancer.

**Li Zhang and Jong Bok Lee:**

Our current research project aims to develop a new immunotherapy using a very small subset of T cell lymphocytes called double-negative T (DNT) cells. Unlike conventional T cells, DNT cells lack surface expression of CD4 and CD8, hence the name.

When cancer cells develop a lot of mutations, they start proliferating rapidly, which causes them to acquire stress-induced ligands. We have determined that DNT cells can recognize these ligands through NKG2D receptors.151 In response, DNT cells release cytotoxic molecules called granzymes and perforin, which puncture holes in target cells, leading to the death of those cells; this is how DNT cells kill cancer cells.

In general, T cells are involved in the anti-cancer response and in fighting viral infections, but can also contribute to graft rejection and autoimmune diseases if they are not well-controlled.

The advantage of DNT cells compared to conventional T cells (which express either CD4 or CD8) is that they do not cause allogeneic reaction. This means that T cells from a donor can be injected into a recipient without the risk of causing graft versus host disease (GvHD).[152]

Our focus is on obtaining DNT cells from healthy donors and utilizing them in the treatment of cancer patients.[151-152] To elaborate, we can expand DNT cells in large numbers and infuse them back into the patient as a way of taking advantage of the strength of the immune system.

# CHAPTER 5: DETECTING AND DIAGNOSING CANCER

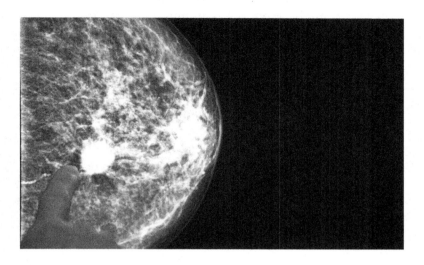

## How are most cancers detected and diagnosed today?

**Josh Ofman:**

We've been fighting a war against cancer for decades. It's not a war we're winning, and that's in large part because the majority of cancers are simply detected too late—after they've already spread.

Currently, there are no early detection methods or screening tests for the deadliest cancers. In the U.S., we screen for five types of cancer: breast, colon, cervical, prostate, and—in high-risk smokers—lung cancer.

Most cancer deaths (70% - 80%) occur as a result of cancers for which there are no available screening methods.[153] These cancers include pancreas, ovary, stomach, head and neck, and liver cancer.

**Jo Bhakdi:**

For most cancers, such as kidney, bladder, pancreatic, and lung cancer, there are no screenings. In theory, there are tools that could be used to screen, but there are no standard-of-care screenings because they yield so many false positives and false negatives.

Some cancers are detected incidentally, such as by MRI or CT for an unrelated problem (e.g., injury from a car accident), but most cancers go completely undetected until it's too late (i.e., when the patient is already symptomatic). One can imagine that the odds of successfully treating cancers that are detected at a late stage are not very high.

For some cancers, such as colon cancer, screenings are recommended every 10 years, but what happens in between screenings? Breast cancer screenings are recommended annually or biannually for women of a certain age, depending on the country. For people who live in very sun-intensive areas, annual skin screenings are recommended, but the screenings themselves are not very effective.[154]

Overall, adherence to the screening guidelines that do exist is only 10% - 20%.

Once cancer has been detected, there's no question that a biopsy is required for a diagnosis. The question is, how do people get to that point? When and how do the red flags emerge and point to the need for further investigation?

**Ruchi Gaba:**

Cancer that is detected in asymptomatic people is often detected incidentally, and this is definitely true when it comes to thyroid cancer. In order to notice a lump in the neck, it has to be at least a centimeter in size (some people will not notice a lump in their neck until it has reached two centimeters in size). Thyroid cancer presenting in this way will not cause any pain and usually won't secrete any excess thyroid hormone—it will just sit there and grow.

Tumors less than a centimeter in size are called micro-cancers or micro-papillary cancers. It's unclear how much clinical significance there is to performing a biopsy on a micro-cancer, because what if, left undisturbed, it would never grow or metastasize?

**Rabia Bhatti:**

When it comes to breast cancer detection, mammography is usually the first step. Mammography uses X-rays to produce images of breast tissue. However, X-rays don't work on dense breast tissue, so we use ultrasound (i.e., sonography) instead. If ultrasound doesn't yield clear images, then we will use MRI. We will also use MRI for patients who have had cancer previously, or who have a strong family history of breast cancer.

We calculate every single patient's risk of developing breast cancer based on what's called a Tyrer-Cuzick score.[155] This is a score that takes into account multiple factors, including family history, the age of the patient at the onset of their first menstrual cycle, and whether the patient has any biological children.

The average U.S. woman's risk of developing breast cancer is about 13%.[156] If we determine that a patient's lifetime risk of developing breast cancer is more than 20%, then we will recommend MRI in addition to a mammogram.

We also have high-risk clinics designed to screen high-risk women at a much earlier age than the recommended age of 40 and above.

**Susan Wadia-Ells:**

About 10,000 women in the U.S. each year who undergo a screening mammography—the primary method for identifying breast irregularities…. heavily promoted by the for-profit cancer industry —are diagnosed with either Stage 0 or Stage 1 breast cancer.[157] These women are told they have early-stage breast cancer, when in fact, those with Stage 0 simply have atypical cells, also called ductal carcinoma in situ (DCIS). They do not have a cancerous tumor. Women diagnosed with a Stage 1 breast tumor usually have pea sized dormant tumors that have existed for decades, and may never actually grow. Treating either of these conditions with biopsies and other invasive cancer protocols can, in fact, stimulate such cells to become cancerous and initiate advanced breast cancer. This is why many researchers now understand that today's mammography industry is simply a feeder system for today's unnecessary breast cancer epidemic.

Many of us have been brainwashed into thinking that mammograms somehow prevent breast cancer, and are terrified by the thought of not having them routinely. But mammograms do not prevent anything. They use toxic radiation to see if you have aypical cells or pea-size tumors so that the breast cancer industry can begin to treat you and increase their profits. Women who have dangerous or fast-growing breast tumors find these tumors themselves.

You can find much more information about today's unnecessary breast cancer epidemic in my recent book, *Busting Breast Cancer: Five Simple Steps to Keep Breast Cancer Out of Your Body.*


**Steve Gullans:**

There is a lot of great innovation on the cancer diagnostics front. Of course, we all understand the value of routine screening with mammography or PSA testing. In addition, once a tumor is known to exit from imaging, obtaining a small piece of a tumor can be very informative, especially in terms of the presence or absence of different immune cells or cancer markers that can predict responsiveness to certain therapies. In addition, recently there has been strong interest in a liquid biopsy, which tests blood, stool, or other bodily fluids for the presence of tumor cells or tumor DNA with certain mutations or marker chromosomes thought to indicate the presence of a tumor.

# The benefits of liquid vs. traditional surgical biopsy

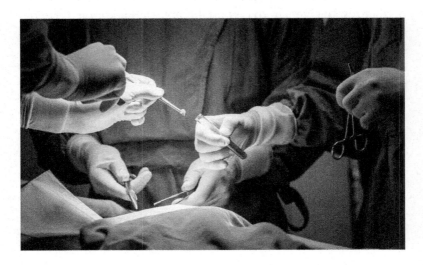

**Josh Ofman:**

The term 'liquid biopsy' was coined to reflect how cancer can be studied by looking at a blood sample instead of a solid tissue sample. The term is now being applied more broadly to mean examining a blood sample for anything related to cancer, regardless of whether there is a diagnosis of cancer. I would prefer that the term 'liquid biopsy' be reserved for cases where the patient is known to have cancer.

The purpose of a liquid biopsy is to examine fragments of DNA circulating in the blood and identify signals of cancer. When liquid biopsy is used in people who have not received a diagnosis of cancer, it's like trying to find a needle in a haystack, from a signal-to-noise ratio standpoint. However, in a patient who is known to have cancer, the signal is incredibly strong and there's not nearly as much noise to contend with.

To put it simply, the technical challenges differ greatly between liquid biopsy done on a person who has cancer and liquid biopsy done on a person who does not have cancer.

**Jo Bhakdi:**

Liquid biopsy will transform the field of cancer diagnostics over the next 10 years. It's a game-changer, because current methods are so bad.

In a liquid biopsy, we look for circulating cell-free DNA fragments, which are DNA fragments that have been shed into the blood by cells that have died. With single-molecule precision, we can identify which fragments of DNA in a blood sample carry tumor variants or mutations.[158]

Why is liquid biopsy such a transformative technology? A liquid biopsy is like obtaining a systemic fingerprint of the tumor as it presents itself as a systemic phenomenon. This is because in the blood, the entire tumor is "mixed up," whereas one sample of a tumor is *not* representative of the systemic presentation of the tumor.[159] In the blood, everything is represented—the heterogeneity of the entire primary tumor, metastases, etc.

The downside of liquid biopsies is that a lower concentration is obtained, which means certain things can't be seen. Nonetheless, it provides a reliable systemic picture of the tumor, which is much more important in terms of chemotherapeutics.

My thesis is that liquid biopsy will be highly beneficial for systemic treatments, because it is a systemic diagnostic as opposed to a tissue biopsy.

**Christos Chinopoulos:**

The liquid biopsy is the next best thing, though it is still in its infancy. One of the main reasons I like it is because it can assist with early cancer detection, and can help patients avoid being subjected to invasive hard tissue biopsies, full-body imaging, etc.

**Jyotsna Batra:**

While liquid biopsy biomarkers can detect with high accuracy the presence of prostate cancer and the predicted probability that a patient will develop a tumor,160 these biomarkers are not good predictors of disease aggressiveness, which is the current problem when it comes to prostate cancer. Even using the PSA (prostate-specific antigen) blood test, we cannot predict whether a tumor is going to be aggressive or non-aggressive.

Liquid biopsy success in this area has been limited by the number of patients which have been analyzed, because 70% - 80% of a patient cohort is going to have non-aggressive, slow-growing prostate cancer. Analysis via liquid biopsy has never been done on a very large cohort, which is likely why we have not been successful.

In addition, tumor heterogeneity plays a huge role, and must be considered.160 Liquid biopsy results need to be identified and interpreted with a lot of caution in this regard, and much more research is needed in the field.

**George Calin**:

The liquid biopsy is an extremely powerful tool. The idea behind it is to identify what is happening at the site of the disease without having to directly access the site of the disease, as doing so can cause harm to the patient.[161-162]

Since tumors release proteins, hormones, and other products into the bloodstream, the liquid biopsy can be used to identify and examine the blood for signs of cancer. Most of the research has been focused on identifying biomarkers in the blood from the spectrum of non-coding RNA (short or long). However, this can also be done using other bodily fluids, such as urine, gastric juice, and cerebrospinal fluid.

# Early detection to improve treatment outcomes

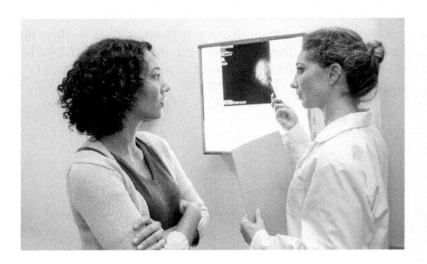

**Andreas Mershin:**

A 2004 paper published in *BMJ* describes how dogs have been trained to diagnose bladder cancer with 41% success (compared to 14% without any training).[163] The success rate would have been even higher had it not been for one sample that the dog kept "misidentifying." It was later discovered that this sample, despite being classified as "clean" in the study, belonged to a patient who indeed had very early-stage bladder cancer—so early that it could not be detected by conventional tests.

I wondered what it is that dogs can detect that even the most advanced tests to date cannot.

In a different study, a dog by the name of Daisy alerted Dr. Claire Guest (by repeatedly nudging her chest) to a very deeply buried breast cancer nodule that was difficult to detect even with mammography. Dr. Guest's doctors informed her that her prognosis could have been quite severe had she not been alerted by Daisy so early on.[164]

But perhaps the most surprising and intriguing part of the story is that Daisy had only been trained to detect bladder cancer—not breast cancer[164]—and the bouquet of volatile organic compounds produced as part of the metabolic activity of each tumor type is completely different. In fact, there are no signature volatiles that identify the presence of cancer in general; for each type of cancer, the list of volatile compounds is different from any and all other types of cancer.[165] Yet, dogs can generalize and find a pattern.

As an analogy, think of the molecules of scent produced by the metabolic pathways as sand, and the cancer signatures like footsteps in the sand. There can be different types of sand in different part of the body, but the signature of cancer is like an imprint in the sand that rides on all of them, yet none of them individually.

We believe that the dog is essentially mining the scent character of cancer,[165] similar to how humans use their noses.

Consider, for example, that when we smell a cup of coffee, we are not analyzing it based on the concentration of different molecules it contains. Olfaction tells us what something smells of, not what it's made of. Similarly, when we look at the Mona Lisa painting, we perceive it all at once—not pixel by pixel.

Cancer manifests itself in many different ways, including by leaving an imprint that is diagnosable by the emergent scent character much more so than by individual molecules. Individual molecules might be different from human to human or from tissue to tissue, but the cancer signature appears to be generalizable, mineable, and quantifiable, at least through the nose of the dog.

Using human urine from consenting adults, we hope to train dogs and machines through AI technology to not only diagnose cancer[165] (which is relatively easy), but to determine the severity of cancer, because this will inform treatment. And in the case of prostate cancer, this can mean the difference between life and death.

For the last 15 to 20 years, we know that dogs have outcompeted machines in terms of their ability to diagnose disease.[166] We want the machines to detect with identical accuracy as dogs, so that dogs and machines are indistinguishable in this regard.

Our group, along with many other groups, have shown that dogs can be pushed to very great limits of detection, and they can also be mimicked by machines using technology that already exists, and that can fit inside a smartphone.[167]

**Christos Chinopoulos:**

Early detection methods are being actively pursued with the use of fluorodeoxyglucose and fluoroglutamine in positron emission tomography/computed tomography (PET/CT). Fluorodeoxyglucose and fluoroglutamine are futile derivatives of glucose and glutamine, respectively.

Cancer cells avidly take up glucose and glutamine in the body, and they do the same with these derivatives. By delivering fluorodeoxyglucose and fluoroglutamine prior to PET/CT imaging, areas of high uptake will light up on the scan, indicating the presence of cancer cells.[168-169]

Metastases of around 105 cancer cells are detectable using this method,170 which is too small to be discernable by the naked eye during a surgical procedure. This method also demonstrates superior detection capability compared to conventional imaging methods.[169]

**Josh Ofman:**

When cancer cells die during the process of growth and invasion, they shed little bits of DNA into the blood. The idea at GRAIL has been to determine the best way to examine that DNA in order to find cancer, which was done through the Circulating Cell-free Genome Atlas (CCGA) study.[171]

This study involved a head-to-head comparison of the value of looking at gene mutations, chromosomal changes, and epigenetic or methylation changes to detect cancer. Using a machine learning algorithm, cancer signals were distinguishable from non-cancer signals based on methylation patterns.[171]

Since then, we've been able to discriminate with very high accuracy cancer signals that are circulating in a person's blood. This technology has the ability to detect cancer in people who do not even know they have it.

GRAIL has pioneered the Galleri™ test, which is a simple blood test that can detect over 50 different types of cancer.[172] The result will state that either no cancer signal was detected, or that a cancer signal was detected. If the latter results, there will be a predicted origin of that cancer signal (e.g., liver, ovary, stomach, or head and neck). This will provide guidance as to where to look for the cancer signal.

We estimate that if we introduced the Galleri™ test into the population, we could intercept about 70% of cancers at a much earlier stage. This could have a dramatic impact on the cancer death rate.

Of those people who are likely to die of cancer within the next five years, data from the U.S. suggests that we could prevent death in 39% of them by simply using the Galleri™ test as an early detection method.[173] To put that number in context, that's about 100,000 deaths averted every year.

This new multi-cancer early detection technology could have a dramatic impact on public health.

**Eric Fung:**

Even the earliest stages of cancer can provide a hallmark of both the presence of cancer as well as where that cancer came from. This is borne out by data from the CCGA study,[171] as well as PATHFINDER, an interventional study that evaluated the clinical integration of a multi-cancer early detection (MCED) blood test.[174]

Solid cancers tend to progress from a precancerous state to invasive cancer, the latter of which we describe as being stage I-IV. Using a targeted methylation approach, the MCED test can detect as early as stage I cancer, and also determine where it came from.[174] This tells us that the molecular hallmarks of cancer are present even at the earliest stages, and we can detect them as long as the tumor DNA shedding rate is high enough.

Some of the types of cancers that will most benefit from early detection include ovarian, pancreatic, esophageal, and liver. Some cancers may be better screened for using other approaches. For example, melanoma can be deadly once it spreads, but since there is already a skin screening test that can be very helpful for early detection, a blood test for melanoma may be of lower value.

**Denis Noble:**

A recent study from University College London scanned the lungs of a large number of people who in no way had any suspicion that they might have lung cancer (i.e., they were completely asymptomatic).[175] The findings showed that lung cancer can be detected very early on, before the person has any sign of it.

This means that routinely scanning people for signs of lung cancer—much in the same way that we do for breast cancer—could lead to very early detection, which would make surgical intervention very effective.

# CHAPTER 6: TREATING CANCER

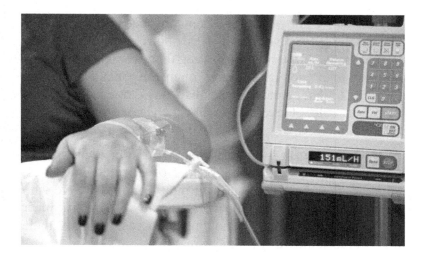

## Is the "gold standard" of cancer treatment effective?

**Gary Foresman:**

The classic saying is that all medicines are poison—it's just a matter of the dosage. This is true for blood pressure medication, cholesterol medication, diabetes medication, etc. The term "chemo" usually refers to cytotoxic chemotherapy, which is medicine that essentially treats growth and is used specifically for cancer.

When a person walks into an MD's office, they are essentially asking for poison, which is something most people don't realize. Cancer specialists are not really cancer specialists; the standard oncologist is a specialist in using poisons to treat cancer, and most of them don't even know about the off-label uses of other forms of chemo (i.e., alternative drugs for cancer treatment). I'm not bagging on chemotherapy specialists; I am simply trying to make the point that they are not cancer specialists.

How do we know this? We know this because they do not address the patient's level of stress, nutrition, or exercise—despite many studies demonstrating that exercise is far more effective than chemotherapy regimens, especially for colon cancer.176 The cancer specialist does not address the important role of exercise because there is no lobby for exercise; there is, of course, a lobby for chemotherapy.

The point I want to make is that Western medicine is of a limited viewpoint in that it focuses on chemotherapeutics, radiation therapy, and/or surgical intervention. Anyone who really looks into all of the data on alternative forms of cancer treatment would realize that not much progress has been made in the "gold standard" of cancer treatment.

The average MD is often looked upon as a high priest or priestess of Western medicine, which is very dangerous, because they use a belief system to treat people; they believe in drugs over all of the other available options for cancer treatment, like exercise and nutrition.

In other parts of the word, people are much more open to other types of therapy. For example, in China, everything from herbs to diets to spiritual practices are considered as possible forms of cancer treatment.

People need to be aware of what the standard of care really is, and they have to be smart enough to know that there are little fragments of truth within it. For instance, statins are effective in secondary prevention of cardiovascular disease, so there is a role for them. But lowering a person's cholesterol level only through the use of drugs is a horrifically bad strategy, yet that's the standard of care.

For decades now, through advertising on TV and other outlets, people have started to believe that the only way to treat any ailment—including cancer—is by taking drugs.

My experience has shown me that the standard of care tells me what I shouldn't be doing.

**Matthew Vander Heiden:**

As an oncologist, I like to remind people that no one wants to receive chemotherapy; it can be tough medicine, but we use it because it works.

Many people who have localized breast cancer undergo surgery and radiation, followed by chemotherapy. The chemotherapy helps fewer people develop the disease again by killing the disease somewhere else in the body.

Chemotherapy often gets a bad name because of the side effects. But cutting through the side effects, the truth is that many cancers have been cured through the use of chemotherapy, including childhood leukemia.

In addition, chemotherapy is often referred to as a nonspecific poison; while some of it certainly is poison, to say that it is nonspecific isn't always fair. For instance, some of the best chemotherapies very specifically target enzymes in particular metabolic pathways.

It is striking that the same drugs that work phenomenally in treating some cancers don't work at all in other cancers. This challenges the notion that chemotherapies only work by attacking all dividing cells. Yes—they do attack dividing cells, which is why they cause hair loss and problems with the gut, but the cells in the gut proliferate much faster than tumor cells. Further, two tumors proliferating at the same rate may respond differently to a particular drug.

All of this indicates that the chemotherapeutic mechanism is not simply a matter of attacking all dividing cells. Instead, we think that certain cancer cells must be more sensitive than normal cells to the enzymes targeted by specific drugs.

**Carlo Maley:**

The standard of care for most cancers is a multidrug cocktail, with each drug executing a different mechanism to kill cells. Some of these cocktails contain as many as four different drugs. This approach works very well for HIV, where we've maintained disease control for decades using a three-drug cocktail.[177]

In cancer biology, it doesn't work nearly as well. Increasing the number of drugs from one to two in the treatment of cancer might buy an extra few months of survival time (or a year for those who are lucky), but adding a third drug has zero effect, according to meta-analyses of lung cancer.[178] One of the issues here is that the toxicity of the drugs adds up, so combining more than two is not effective.

If a tumor could be sequenced and the dominant clones identified, then it might be possible to find one drug that could target each clone. The challenge is that in many cases, the cells that are resistant to a drug are so rare that they won't be identified through sequencing analysis of a solid tissue sample.[179] There could be one drug-resistant cancer cell in a million or even a billion other cells, so this strategy can be very challenging.

**David Goode:**

Different regions of a tumor may be genetically and molecularly different, which has big implications for drug resistance[179]; one part of the tumor might respond really well to the drug, shrink, and die off, while another part may be completely resistant to the drug, and therefore grow back.

The problem is that with traditional biopsies, just one small sample of tissue is obtained from the overall tumor, which could be quite large. This means that information about the rest of the tumor—indeed the majority of the tumor—will be missed.[180] Often, people are misled into thinking that the tissue sample used for biopsy is genetically and molecularly representative of the *entire* tumor. As a result, important clues about the best way to treat the patient easily go missed.

**Thomas Seyfried:**

A young man who had glioblastoma and paralysis on his entire left side was put on metabolic therapy for three weeks prior to a debulking surgery. He was doing so well that radiation therapy was postponed for three months, which is unheard of in the oncology field. However, he was pressured into receiving massive doses of radiation.

"Why are you doing this?" I asked the oncologist. "This guy is doing really well. He's healthy right now." The oncologist maintained his position, and radiation treatment began. He survived radiation treatment and the chemotherapy drug temozolomide—so-called standard-of-care measures.

After 24 months, the patient was still in pretty good health, but then he began developing headaches and died quickly thereafter. The autopsy showed necrosis and massive radiation damage to his brain; in essence, his brain had been liquified by the radiation.

Is that ethical? Is it ethical to irradiate someone's brain until it liquefies?

I'm not opposed to radiation therapy for every kind of cancer. In fact, if there is evidence that radiation therapy can provide 90% or better recovery and management of the disease, then go for it. But to nuke someone who has glioblastoma or another type of advanced cancer is fundamentally unethical.

**Josh Ofman:**

There is a common misperception in the population, which is that most cancers don't have an effective treatment. But in fact, most solid tumors in the early localized stage are eminently treatable and often curable with surgery and radiation—we just don't hear this often because not many cases of cancer are caught early enough.

Many cases of breast cancer are being cured because we tend to detect breast cancer early. The same is true for colon, cervical, prostate, and lung cancer.

**Samantha Bucktrout:**

We are finding that different chemotherapies have different impacts on the immune response; some chemotherapies are thought to have negative impacts on the immune system, but some could potentially have positive impacts on the immune system.[181] For example, some chemotherapies can actually open up the tumor microenvironment and allow the immune system to be activated in that space.

Clinical successes are coming from a combination of chemotherapy and immunotherapy, which has been a welcome surprise to immunologists. Going forward, the goal is to figure out why this combination is effective, and how to better understand and implement chemotherapies.

**Ruchi Gaba:**

When it comes to thyroid cancer, surgery is the main modality, followed by radioactive iodine given in the form of a pill. Iodine is one of the main substrates for hormone production, and the thyroid cells will be hungry for it; the idea is that the radioactive iodine will kill the remaining thyroid cells that consume it.

Most patients do really well with surgery and radioactive iodine, but in rare cases of advanced thyroid cancer or metastases, tyrosine kinase inhibitors may be used.[182] Chemotherapy is a last resort that sometimes becomes necessary.

**Kornelia Polyak:**

Almost half of the patients who have triple-negative breast cancer are cured by chemotherapy alone, with recurrence happening in these patients only very rarely. In contrast, patients with hormone receptor-positive disease in general respond well to hormone therapy, but will often have late recurrence.

Whether chemotherapy will be an effective treatment depends in part upon the type of tumor. For instance, HER2-targeted therapy can be very effective, but within a HER2-positive tumor, there may be a fraction of cells that lack HER2.[183] Since chemotherapy is less biased than targeted therapy (i.e., it targets proliferating cells as opposed to a specific target), it may be more effective in treating some HER2-positive tumors in combination with HER2-targeting agents.

That said, chemotherapy certainly shouldn't be given to people who are unlikely to respond well to it, because there are obvious side effects.

Our goal is to match patients with the best therapeutic approach at any given time, because even the same patient may require different therapies depending on the stage of disease progression or recurrence.

# Can chemotherapy and/or radiation cause tumor recurrence?

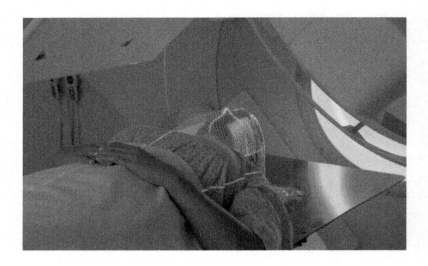

**Carlo Maley:**

I'm very interested in everything that occurs at the intersection of cancer and evolution.

Within our body, cells are evolving, mutating, and competing—particularly in tumors. Some of these mutations can cause a cancer or precancerous cell to divide faster or survive better than its competitors, and those mutant cells will tend to grow.

A microcosm of natural selection happens in our bodies and drives the process of cancer development, and when we apply therapy to this process, we end up applying selective pressure to the tumor. In other words, we kill many of the cancer cells using chemotherapies, but we simultaneously select for mutants that are resistant to those chemotherapies.

Those mutations occur by chance. There are billions of cells in a tumor and millions of mutations, so it is quite common for a mutation to—by chance—show resistance to chemotherapy, and therefore survive.

The whole process of natural selection occurring at the cellular level explains both how we get cancer and why it's been so hard to cure.

**Perry Marshall:**

There are two terms that apply here: monoclonal and multiclonal.

In this context, monoclonal means that the cancer cells are derived from one cancer cell and are all the same, more or less. This would typically be seen in an early-stage tumor, where a cell or group of cells has gone rogue, and their progeny are clones of the original cell.

Multiclonal, on the other hand, means there are multiple species of cancer present—like a mixture of dogs, cats, zebras, corn plants, rabbits, etc.

When an oncologist performs a biopsy of a tumor, they will determine the monoclonality of the cells they see. In other words, they will determine that all the cancer cells are basically alike and will choose a treatment designed to kill those types of cells. They may be right or wrong about that, but the point is that it's still one species of cancer—like all rabbits or all cats or all zebras.

Many times, chemotherapy and aggressive treatments push monoclonal populations of cells into massive evolutionary proliferation. In other words, a population that starts as all rabbits will evolve within 30 to 60 days into a population containing muskrats, squirrels, gerbils, rats, mice, etc. And at that point, no one will have any idea how to kill *all* of those species, especially considering that they each have different abilities and methods of adaptation.

**Kenneth Pienta:**

A few years ago while studying the microenvironment of cancers by creating artificial cancer on a chip, we discovered the poly-aneuploid cancer cell, which is really a state that cancer cells go through when they're subjected to stress.[184] For instance, cancer cells in a primary tumor can get stressed due to low oxygen levels.

We found that when treating a tumor with chemotherapy, the majority of cells die, but a subset of poly-aneuploid cells double their DNA (get stronger), which allows them to find resistance mutations.

In addition, they hibernate like sleeping bears and stop proliferating while the stress is around.[185] This makes it so that chemotherapy cannot kill them, since chemotherapy works by killing proliferating cells. Once there are no more chemotherapy drugs in the system, the poly-aneuploid cells repopulate the tumor with many new resistant cancer cells.[185]

We also found that even while hibernating, these cells can actually move around the body, thereby causing the cancer to spread.[185] The poly-aneuploid cancer cell explains resistance and why we have been unable to cure cancer.

**Denis Noble:**

During late-stage metastasis, there is rapid mutation (also referred to as hypermutation). When we zap people with radiotherapy and use chemotherapy, we risk the development of new genetic mutations that will be even more resistant to the treatment.

Even if surgery, radiotherapy, or chemotherapy initially succeeded in shrinking a tumor or making it apparently disappear, metastatic cancer can return two or three years later. Presumably, this is because a small minority of cells became resistant to treatment due to having developed certain mutations during the period of rapid mutation.

Since there isn't a central controller in terms of which cells will develop resistance, the cancer that recurs years later often won't be genetically identical to the original cancer.

**Adrienne C. Scheck:**

There are studies that show that some chemotherapies promote more genetic instability,[186] but not necessarily a specific mutation. In other words, therapy is not going to drive the tumor in a particular direction.

What can be said is that certain therapies can kill cells with certain behaviors, and the cells that are left are resistant to that therapy. This means that it's not a matter of driving the occurrence of a specific mutation as much as it is selecting for cells with a specific mutation by killing off the vast majority of cells.

In brain tumors, chemotherapy and radiation kills the majority of the cells, but leaves some resistant cells. Once those chemo-resistant cancer cells begin growing, genetic heterogeneity returns.

It is kind of like playing whack-a-mole, but if enough moles can be eliminated, it may be possible to determine what it is about those cells that makes them resistant to chemotherapy.

**Christos Chinopoulos:**

A well-known problem in certain cancers is the recurrence of a second tumor following chemotherapy. However, the second tumor will look quite different from the first.

For example, in breast cancer, a primary tumor may respond well to a certain chemotherapeutic regimen. However, after a year or two, the patient will develop another tumor that will not respond to that same regimen.

By sequencing the second tumor, it will be shown that it does not use the same genes as the original tumor that was treated. In these cases, the primary tumor has learned to become immune to the weapon of choice—that weapon being chemotherapy.

How the tumor does this is unbelievable, and it's not by mistake or error; it is the ability to adapt to chemotherapeutic agents through a process that might rightly be named the evolution of cancer.

# How can cancer be treated immunologically?

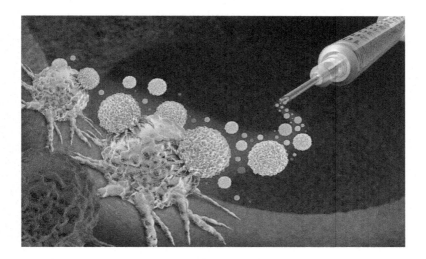

**Samantha Bucktrout:**

Immunotherapy engages with the immune system, which is the body's natural clearing house for cancer. Through the process of cell division, potentially precancerous and cancer cells are produced every day; it is the job of the immune system to detect and eliminate those cells.

When the standard of care (i.e., surgery, chemotherapy, radiation) results in poor outcomes, it's usually because the cancer itself is actively blocking the immune system. Cancer is able to do this because it is part of our body, and our body has a natural ability to regulate the immune system.

Immunotherapies have been successful up until now based on our understanding of the barriers that cancer puts up. Since we know what those barriers are, we can block them with proteins, antibodies, and large molecules.

These therapies have given patients long-lasting disease control, extending lives beyond 10 years and improving quality of life. In some patients—even those who had metastatic disease that is usually fatal—the word "cure" can be used following successful immunotherapy, which is really exciting.

**Kenneth Pienta:**

From an immune system standpoint, the most important part of fighting cancer is the presence of cytotoxic T cells that can attack the tumor. These cytotoxic T cells are supported by antitumorigenic M1 macrophages (macrophages that are helpful in fighting cancer) as opposed to protumorigenic M2 macrophages.[122]

The problem is that when we immunosuppress someone, we suppress everything. In other words, there is no way to selectively suppress M2 macrophages, but keep cytotoxic T cells working. This is where checkpoint inhibitor-based immunotherapy comes into play; the idea behind it is to selectively turn on cytotoxic T cells and enhance the immune system.[187]

**Carlo Maley:**

One of the big breakthroughs in cancer therapy has involved the ability to interfere with mechanisms of immune system evasion by cancer cells. In other words, the goal is to help the immune system regain the ability to detect and attack cancer cells.

This can be accomplished by interfering with the signals at two main immune checkpoints: cytotoxic T-lymphocyte-associated antigen 4 (CTLA-4) and programmed death 1 (PD-1).[188] By blocking these checkpoints, the immune system can begin to recognize the tumor again.

However, since there are multiple mechanisms for immune system evasion by cancer cells, a tumor will evolve other ways to get around the immune system. For this reason, these immune-based therapies work only some of the time, and in many cases, the patient will relapse with a tumor that has a different phenotype for immune system evasion.

**Richard White III:**

Immunotherapy can involve infecting tumor cells with a virus, which would lead to the production of molecules on the surface of the tumor cells, which would trigger cytotoxic T cell activity. An important distinction here is that the virus is not necessarily being used to kill tumor cells, but to infect them so that the immune system can recognize and eradicate the cancer cells.

Vesicular stomatitis virus (VSV) is a rhabdovirus that's been used as a potential way of killing tumor cells, and it is thought that it could potentially attack inoperable brain tumors.[189]

Another idea is to use mRNA from a virus to specifically target tumor cells. The mRNA would be taken in by the tumor cells, and would then make several proteins which would alert the cytotoxic T cells to their presence. The T cells would then be able to destroy the tumor.

I think the sky is the limit—we just have to be careful to target the right cells and leave the healthy ones unaffected.

**Brendon Coventry:**

We have had recent successes using a cancer vaccine therapy for curing advanced cancer. Patients with advanced melanoma have survived for over 20-years with vaccine therapy alone and this is currently being developed and commercialised (Cancuravax Ltd) for patient usage, and this may likely extend to other cancer types. Further development of these techniques are underway. Historically, there have been many recorded successes (i.e., improved outcomes, decreased chances of recurrence) with 'neoadjuvant therapies' (neo = new, adjuvant = help) - immunotherapy[189-190], and other therapies (chemotherapies and radiation therapies) which are delivered prior to surgery as opposed to adjuvant treatments, which are delivered following surgery (to help stop the resected cancer coming back).

This demonstrates that boosting the immune system prior to surgical removal of a tumor may eliminate the need for surgery, because the tumor could disappear altogether, or to the point that only a small amount of scarring remains. The problem is that this isn't always the result; a tumor may persist despite neoadjuvant treatment and surgery will still be required. It is not a 'one-size-fits-all' approach.

Although immune therapies of many types (e.g., Tuberculosis vaccines, other bacterial products) have been used partially successfully for treatment of cancer by those pioneers exploring immune treatments[247], perhaps one of the most instructive is the first US FDA approved treatment, Interleukin-2 (IL-2), which is one of the natural drivers of immune cells (T-cells) causing them to divide and become activated, promoting the anti-cancer immune response[247,253] and even most importantly producing complete regression of all cancer in some patients (Complete Responses)[254,253].

Anti-programmed death receptors (anti-PD1 receptors) are often used as neoadjuvant therapies (trade names include nivolumab and pembrolizumab). These therapies prevent the death of lymphocytes by blocking the death receptor that, when activated, contributes to lymphocyte cell death.[191] This prolongs the life of immune cells close to the tumor. Another treatment which has proved effective is anti-CTLA4 (Cytotoxic T-Lymphocyte Associated protein-4) receptor therapies, which effectively take the 'brakes' off of the T-cell immune response, to release the inhibition of T-lymphocytes to activate them against the cancer[247]. Indeed, complete response (CR) have been reported with anti-CTLA4 agents. The combination of both anti-PD1 and anti-CTLA4 agents have been even more effective in inducing CRs, but at the cost of 'auto-immunity' where the patient's own normal tissues are attacked causing sometimes major side-effects, including death in some 1-2% of cases. Most interestingly, the incidence of auto-immune side-effects is also associated with the effectiveness against the tumor[247].

These therapies can be used on both liquid (blood, leukemias) and solid (main tumor types involving solid organs) tumors, because they bind to PD-1 (programmed cell death protein 1) on lymphocytes that are close to or capable of infiltrating the tumor, which means they are related to the immune system and not necessarily the tumor cells themselves.

Also, most fascinatingly, the microbial population present in the patient's gut at the time of treatment has been shown to influence the effectiveness of the immune checkpoint treatment (anti-PD1 and anti-CTLA4). Further, this has even been more specifically localised to several species of bacteria being present or absent in the gut microflora or microbiota [255,247,248,256]. Perhaps unsurprisingly from this information, antibiotic therapy can influence the effectiveness of ICI immunotherapy. The immune response is becoming even more influential in determining the survival outcome from cancer immunotherapy - a fact that is of outstanding immunological significance which we must understand better.

Chimeric T-cell antigen (CAR-T) therapies utilise laboratory re-engineered T-cells (ex-vivo; outside the patient) that have the ability to react with cancer associated antigens extracted from the cancer.

A small group of cancer associated T-cells, inside the patient are already 'seeing' tumour antigens. By designing T-cells with receptors for those similar antigens in the laboratory and infusing those back into the patient, the immune response against the cancer can be enhanced or boosted resulting in effective tumour removal. This is both an interesting and novel treatment, but it is currently complicated and relatively expensive, however, most importantly it proves that T-cells of the correct type can eliminate cancer cells.

It is my belief that most, if not all, cancer therapies are actually manipulating the patient's own immune system to produce either an 'effective' or 'ineffective' immune responses and thereby either 'cure' or 'failure', or something 'in-between'. This means that the different treatments causing the killing or the damaging of cancer cells are actually 'vaccinating' the cancer patient against their own cancer, by releasing cancer associated antigens (proteins & lipids) priming their own immune systems to fight the cancer. The reasoning for this view is explained and expanded in detail, as referenced.[247,248] We are actively working on this prospect and are gradually changing some traditional thinking about the effectiveness of 'therapeutic cancer vaccines' for more effectively treating cancer. We are introducing the concept of re-engineering the patient's own immune system to fight their own cancer in-vivo. Multiple therapies such as anti-PD1, anti-CTLA-4, IL-2 and CAR-T cell therapies have shown effectiveness through boosting the pre-existing immune response that is already going on in the patient. Most of these therapies act by 'driving-on' the existing partially effective T-cell immune response, through making it more effective. This approach is proven by the strong evidence of therapeutically vaccinating patients against their own cancer being capable of inducing complete removal of all detectable cancer and long-term survivals of over 20 years, so far.[258,259]

**Herbert Levine:**

The cancer community has become very gung-ho about applying immune system ideas to cancer, because the immune system offers the possibility of outsmarting cancer cells in a way that drugs cannot.

To elaborate, cancer cells are very adaptive, to the point that they often find pathways for defeating drugs—even those administered as part of targeted therapy (which was supposed to defeat cancer 20 years ago). Targeted therapy can prolong lives and it is great to have as an option, but it doesn't really defeat cancer; cancers come back and defeat these drugs instead.

The immune system, on the other hand, is smarter than any non-living drug, because it too is very adaptive. The idea has been to convince the immune system to recognize the tumor as being foreign in the same way that it would recognize a virus as such. Hopefully, with some help, the immune system will recognize tumor cells as foreign and induce immune mechanisms to kill those tumor cells.

It's remarkable that for some subsets of tumors, immune therapies seem to offer the possibility of a cure, meaning no tumor recurrence. But in the case of melanoma, the immunological approach has been shown to work in 10% - 20% of patients,[193] and no one has any idea why it doesn't work in the other 80% - 90%.

To train the immune system to kill any type of cancer cell seems to be a potential cure for cancer, because any time a cancer cell re-emerges and tries to begin growing again, the immune system will be prepared to kill it. In other words, it is possible for someone to become forever immune to whatever caused their cells to become cancerous.

We believe there is a great opportunity to try to understand how different tumor cell behaviors affect interactions with the immune system. Perhaps we can find ways of giving the immune system various boosts in order to defeat a wider range of tumor cell behaviors.

**Doru Paul:**

Over the last decade, checkpoint inhibitors have progressively occupied center stage in oncology and now, these agents are included in the majority of cancer treatment protocols; I think this trend will continue for at least five more years, through the second wave of immunotherapy, which will combine checkpoint inhibitors with other immune system modulators. Ultimately, I believe novel immunotherapy combinations will be discovered and will become new standards of care.

# Treating cancer metabolically

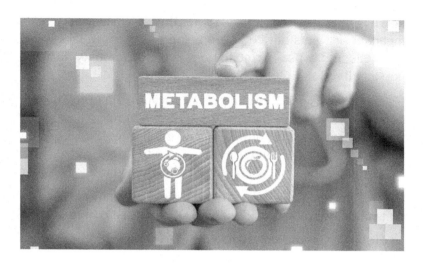

**Thomas Seyfried:**

In the clinic, expensive and elaborate procedures are being used to kill cancer cells, such as CAR T-cell immunotherapy and anti-PD-L1 immunotherapy; these are complicated and sophisticated methods that, in my opinion, are largely unnecessary.

If we can kill cancer cells in a simpler way, without using toxins nor harming the body, then we should. And we can, with a clear and simple metabolic approach to cancer treatment backed by hard science.

If a person holds their breath for long enough, their face will start turning blue, but they won't drop dead instantly. This is because fermentation (the conversion of glucose to energy in the absence of oxygen) can keep our cells alive for a short period of time. However, it is an inefficient process because it causes lactic acid levels in the blood to rise very quickly (this is what causes the skin to appear blue).

Ultimately, a lack of oxygen will quickly cause death. This explains why cyanide kills people so quickly: It shuts down oxidative phosphorylation almost instantly, which means it prevents our cells from using oxygen. In this state, the cells must use fermentation, which can only keep a person alive for so long.

Tumor cells can live and grow in cyanide just fine, which demonstrates that they use fermentation. And since fermentation requires glucose and glutamine, cancer cells require glucose and glutamine in order to stay alive despite a complete shutdown of oxidative phosphorylation.[25]

This means that in order to kill cancer cells, all we have to do is target glucose and glutamine. It's not that complicated.

However, glutamine is an extremely valuable amino acid, so targeting it must be done very strategically with the use of drugs. If glutamine is targeted too aggressively or without an understanding of the biology behind the problem, significant harm can be done to the gut and immune system.

To elaborate, when cancer cells are killed in large numbers, it's the immune system that comes in and cleans up the dead cells in the microenvironment. If glutamine is used in the wrong way, those dead cells persist in the microenvironment, leading to all kinds of adverse consequences.

With a thorough understanding of this, it's not very complicated to kill cancer cells. Yet, the majority of people aren't aware of this.

Metabolic therapy can shrink a tumor to the point that it can be debulked completely, or to the point that it disappears entirely and surgery is not necessary. Why put patients at risk by performing invasive biopsies—procedures which in and of themselves can lead to the spread of the cancer?

A popular argument is that obtaining a tissue sample is necessary in order to examine the gene expression profile and identify which mutations are present prior to delivering chemotherapy and radiation. I argue that mutations are irrelevant; they are downstream epiphenomena that don't mean anything at all, because if we pull the plug on glucose and glutamine, the cancer cell dies and the mutations become entirely irrelevant.

So, why are big companies making billions of dollars by analyzing gene profiles on tissue samples? None of that is necessary. Eliminate the glucose and glutamine, and we eliminate that whole field of oncology.

When it comes to the metabolic approach to cancer treatment, there is tremendous interest on the part of physicians from all over the world who are on the front lines, treating patients firsthand. They want to see people get healthy—that's why they took on the profession they did. They see the value of the metabolic approach I'm explaining here, and they want to know more about it.

The problem is that many physicians who would like to use metabolic therapy are not yet trained to do so properly, and the system is not set up to allow them to learn. If they were to implement therapies that are not sanctioned by the American Medical Association, they would lose their license to practice medicine.

Some physicians would never want to use metabolic therapy simply because it might interfere with their salary. Hospitals are in the business of generating revenue, and metabolic therapy will not generate the same amount of revenue as other therapies. But the truth is that when metabolic therapy is used, a terminal cancer patient can survive up to four times longer than predicted under the standard treatment protocol.[194] And that's the goal.

**Abdul Slocum:**

Having spent over 30 years following and practicing the standard of care in cancer treatment, my two colleagues, Bulent Berkarda and Mehmet Salih İyikesici, and I have seen the shortcomings of it. While researching ways to improve patient outcomes, we stumbled upon hyperthermia, hyperbaric oxygen therapy, and other metabolic therapies.

Hyperthermia treatment has a direct cytotoxic effect by exploiting the heat sensitivity of cancer cells by increasing the main tumor tissue temperature to 42 °C or higher. It also increases the efficacy of most chemotherapeutic agents and radiotherapy.[195]

Many studies have shown that tumor hypoxia is a primary reason some tumors are resistant to chemotherapy and radiotherapy.[196-198] Hyperbaric oxygen therapy targets cancer cells by increasing oxidative stress, which in turn, disrupts this resistance.

Several publications discuss the benefits of combining hyperthermia and hyperbaric oxygen therapy. Aside from having therapeutic effects when used alone, both hyperthermia and hyperbaric oxygen therapy work synergistically with and improve the efficacy of most conventional therapies.[199]

We apply these treatments concomitantly with conventional chemotherapy treatment. We apply chemotherapeutic drugs based on the guidelines, but we use a modified application method which we named metabolically-supported chemotherapy.

In accordance with this application method, patients come to the clinic in a fasting state, having fasted for a minimum of 14 hours. Based on their blood sugar level, we'll apply insulin to cause mild hypoglycemia prior to chemotherapy application, because this causes acute metabolic stress on the cancer cells, weakening them prior to chemotherapy application.

In addition to hyperthermia and hyperbaric oxygen therapy, we often apply the ketogenic diet and some other infusion-based therapies. Our main requirement for any therapy we apply is that it is evidence-based.

Since 2010, we've made eight publications evaluating our treatment outcomes. We have found that combinatorial treatment leads to a significant increase in survival times for many different types of cancer,[200-202] as well as higher quality of life for patients. In addition to being more effective, combinatorial treatment is more tolerable compared to the standard of care.[203]

**Dominic D'Agostino:**

There needs to be a whole new class of oncologist called the metabolic oncologist. Diet should be a cornerstone metabolic therapy, but there's a whole toolbox of metabolic drugs being developed, which are far less damaging to the patient's long-term health than chemotherapy drugs, which wipe out the immune system and make patients more susceptible to developing other forms of cancer. Chemotherapy drugs might extend a patient's life by a couple of months, but will not increase the chances of long-term survival.

As a tumor grows, the biomass of the tumor grows to the point that the blood vessels can't supply enough nutrients and oxygen to the center of the tumor. As a result, the center of the tumor becomes hypoxic, and this hypoxia further damages the mitochondria and impairs oxidative phosphorylation.

The delivery of hyperbaric oxygen to a person causes the plasma portion of the blood to become saturated with oxygen. This not only reverses tumor hypoxia, which could help silence some of the oncogenes and increase tumor suppressor gene activation, but also—and most importantly—causes an oxidative burst inside the tumor itself. This means that the cancer cells will overproduce oxygen free radicals relative to the healthy tissue surrounding it. More or less, the result is a site-specific overproduction of oxygen free radicals.

This is important, especially in the context of other therapies. For example, chemotherapies that work through an oxidative stress mechanism can be augmented by hyperbaric oxygen therapy.[204-205] Further, the efficacy of radiation therapy is directly proportional to the partial pressure of oxygen ($pO_2$) inside the tumor. This means that elevating $pO_2$ inside a tumor will further sensitize that tumor to radiation therapy,[206] which in turn, means that far less radiation is required (about 5% of the normal amount).

When it comes to the metabolic approach to cancer *prevention*, the idea is to have robust metabolic health through anaerobic exercise.[207] I'm a big believer in strength training. This is because skeletal muscle mass dictates mitochondrial health, since building strong and healthy muscles makes the body very hunger for glucose and decreases inflammation. People should focus on optimizing their metabolic health, because metabolic health equals cancer prevention and cancer suppression.

**László Boros:**

The research of Otto Warburg showed that the product of glucose metabolism in cancer cells is lactate, even in the presence of oxygen.[101] This requires mitochondrial dysfunction, because if there are sufficient levels of oxygen and the mitochondria are working properly, then ATP will result via oxidative phosphorylation, and the amount of lactate produced in the process will not be nearly as high as the amount produced by cancer cells.

This was a very significant discovery by Warburg, who later received a Nobel Prize for his discoveries. However, Warburg did not know exactly what type of mitochondrial damage cancer cells suffer (or why, for that matter).

Part of my work has involved clarifying how and why mitochondria become broken in tumor cells. The answer involves the presence of an isotope of hydrogen called deuterium, which is twice as heavy and twice as large as hydrogen in its atomic nucleus.

The problem is that the deuterium nucleus called deuteron breaks the ATP synthase nanomotors in mitochondria, which results in metabolic crowding and excess lactate production. Under normal circumstances, ATP synthase nanomotors in healthy mitochondria rotate 10,000 to 20,000 times per minute and are responsible for transferring hydrogen protons into the mitochondrial matrix (the innermost part of the mitochondrion as well as our body). Deuterium-free water is produced in the matrix as a result.

A number of peer-reviewed papers in the medical literature describe this process.[208-209] The first studies were carried out in the 1980s and showed that when heart muscle is treated with deuterium-containing water, the nanomotors break down and ATP synthesis decreases linearly in the mitochondria of the heart muscle cells.[210]

The body is constantly trying to get rid of deuterium as fast as possible, but once a certain threshold is exceeded, the body becomes overloaded and cannot sufficiently eliminate deuterium before it reaches the mitochondria.

Over time, if enough mitochondria suffer, DNA becomes unstable and aneuploidy (the presence of an abnormal number of chromosomes with irregular DNA content in a cell) can result, which is a key characteristic of cancer cells. These cells then proliferate in an unlimited manner, and that's what cancer is.

To fix this, it's necessary to eliminate deuterium from the diet, and for our cells to consume natural fats instead of processed carbohydrates (sugars), as the former have very low levels of deuterium and the latter have very high levels of deuterium.[211] This can be accomplished through a natural ketogenic diet (https://link.springer.com/content/pdf/10.1007/s11306-021-01855-7.pdf), along with consumption of deuterium-depleted water. We recommend that patients and doctors incorporate deuterium depletion (deupletion) in cancer treatment protocols, regardless of whether they are also delivering radiation, chemotherapy, or other therapies.

**George Yu:**

First let me make it clear that as a surgical oncologist for 35 years, I believe successful treatment of cancer must be a "Cocktail" of approaches and one important intervention is taking advantage of the cancer abnormal mitochondrial function. For the clinical management of cancer patients, we combine a multiple prong intervention.

The analogy I use is in war, you must use different methods to weaken the enemy- starvation, disease, adverse climate, shortage of weapons etc.

- mitochondrial metabolism nutrition CRONK,
- then add on metabolic agents such as dichloroacetate, deoxyglucose and 3 Bromopyruvate etc.,
- incorporate "Repurposed Drugs" such as Metformin, anti-inflammatory drugs, antibiotics, statin drugs etc.
- and use Metronomic low constant dosing chemotherapy and immune drugs, etc.

We know 90% of cancers of all types feed on sugars and carbohydrates using a process called Glycolysis. Cancer metabolism is 60% in the cell cytoplasm and 40% within abnormal the abnormal organelle mitochondria. PET scans fused with CAT scans using FDG a look-alike sugar shows you how active the cancer is eating sugars.

You can empower the patient use CRONK diet or calorie restriction optimal nutrition ketosis to starve the cancer cells.

When you cut sugars out, your body automatically switches to using an alternative energy source from fatty acids called "ketosis". So the patients now can participate in their own care by cutting out sugar and carbohydrates substituting to another food (fuel) using medium chain fatty acids such as coconut oil and eating lots of highly nutritious foods and switch to body ketosis which is good for the rest of the body but the cancer cannot use fatty acids in the beginning. Calorie restriction (1800 calories) has been scientifically shown to promote health and longevity by reversing gene expression even within 2 weeks and arresting chronic diseases such as cancers for over 70 years. The body can undergo autophagy of our "senile cells" when there is insufficient food source.

My late colleague, friend and patient Doctor Richard Veech dedicated his career studying metabolism of the Krebs Cycle with Doctor Hans Krebs and later with Doctor George Cahill to find an alternative fuel from sugars- Ketone esters. At the NIH he replicated the end product of ketosis D Beta Hydroxybutyrate ketone ester- you can even buy it today! The heart and the brain love this ketone ester so does the rest of your body except the cancer cells. Whether you choose Calorie Restriction, fasting in any form, or a ketogenic diet, the end product is this ketone ester as your substitute fuel in place of sugar and carbohydrates.

I'm a surgeon and believe in surgery as part of the treatment debulking the large mass of cancer burden. As early as the 1990s, I believe you must combine many forms of treatments without compromising the patients' immune and endocrine integrity. The answer is a combination of surgery, metabolic therapy, chemotherapy, and radiation...a tailor-made cocktail for the individual patient.[261,262,263,264,265]

**Adrienne C. Scheck:**

We've found that the production of ketones through the ketogenic diet seems to make radiation and chemotherapy more effective in the treatment of brain cancer.[213]

For example, bevacizumab is a drug commonly sold under the brand name Avastin that is designed to reduce angiogenesis. The ketogenic diet reduces the receptor of the molecule rather than the molecule itself, which can improve the efficacy of Avastin. In addition, preliminary experiments suggest that ketones slow the repair of radiation-induced damage to cancer cells.[214]

Ketones are also thought to reduce the invasiveness of tumors. In one extremely metastatic VM mouse model, ketones were shown to reduce the spread and invasiveness of the tumor.[215]

If the vascularization of a tumor can be reduced at the same time that the tumor's ability to spread is reduced, then the therapies that are already being used can be made more effective. In some ways, it could be like a one-two punch.

Experiments using mouse models and cells in culture have demonstrated that the ketogenic diet affects cancer cells in a very different way than it affects normal cells. For instance, it inhibits cancer cell growth, but does not seem to inhibit the growth of normal cells. In fact, normal cells use ketones for energy very well, whereas cancer cells do not.[214]

Although there are no clinical trials demonstrating that the ketogenic will always work to extend a patient's life, there are enough case studies to suggest that it often does. I have heard from a number of people that it seems to help their quality of life and cognition.

That said, it depends on who is being asked and how well they are actually following a ketogenic diet, which is something that should be done with the guidance of a nutritionist or a dietitian who has experience with the ketogenic diet. Some people enter a state of ketosis very easily, while others struggle.

There are many unanswered questions on this topic, but I have seen the ketogenic diet enhance quality of life and increase lifespan for many people.

**Gary Foresman:**

Within the field of natural medicine, there is a basic tenet that nutrition treats people—not diseases. This is something I try to emphasize, because many people assume there is one diet for heart disease, another for cancer, etc. But this assumption overlooks a critical point, which is that it's about the diet that is best for the individual who has the disease—not the disease itself.

Consider the idea of using the ketogenic diet for everyone who has cancer, regardless of their history or dietary approach. For example, if it were recommended for a person who has been on a vegan diet their whole life and who would be stressed about the type of food required for the ketogenic diet, then the stress of making a radical change to their diet could actually make them worse. The same is true when it comes to macrobiotics; macrobiotics help some people, but can kill others because of the stress factor.

What all of this means is that each person should be seen as their own clinical research trial.

When it comes to breast cancer (the type of cancer I see most often), I ask patients about their stress level, how they are coping with their stress, and where they think their cancer has come from.

I start with basic paleo principles, because paleo diets are very straightforward. Humans should eat like humans, which means avoiding processed and inflammatory foods, and getting carbohydrates from organic fruits and vegetables. Together, these dietary changes offer everyone great benefits, including the ability to fight off cancer by boosting immune system function.

Now, I began by explaining the importance of treating the person and not the disease. But this is not universally true, because the more serious and progressed a disease, the more important it becomes to treat the disease—not the person.

Think about it this way: If someone's heart stops beating, we don't ask them about their body type before performing CPR. In other words, we immediately treat the disease in order to have a chance at saving the person, because at such a dire stage, the history of the individual becomes more or less irrelevant.

This brings me to the topic of the ketogenic diet. Is it right for everyone who has cancer? Some would say yes, but for the reasons I've explained here, I would say no. However, I would say that it is great for every person who has late-stage cancer, because the cancer will have reached a degree of seriousness that warrants treatment of the disease, not the person.

**Rabia Bhatti:**

I am a practicing surgeon who has developed a passion for understanding how nutrition and exercise can be used in the prevention and treatment of breast cancer. I believe that exercise is a significant aspect of breast cancer treatment—one that until recently has not be emphasized.

A study published in *Cancers* in May of 2020 showed that women who exercised for two and a half hours per week (the federal guidelines for exercise) had a 60% lower risk of dying of breast cancer and more than 50% lower risk of cancer recurrence,[216] which are tremendous numbers. I am now using exercise as a treatment modality for my patients, and encouraging them to exercise even before treatment has started.

In addition, I obtain the BMI of all of my patients because we know that there is greater risk of cancer recurrence in women with a high BMI.[217] These patients will be referred to one of our dieticians, who primarily recommend the

Mediterranean diet, as it is easier to follow than the ketogenic diet (for patients who prefer the ketogenic diet, we can guide them through it).

Studies have shown that women who practice intermittent fasting have a much lower risk of developing breast cancer, so we will discuss it as a preventive measure once treatment has been completed. We do not usually recommend intermittent fasting while starting treatment for breast cancer because we need patients to be optimized in terms of their nutrition and protein status, and we do not want them to get dehydrated.

**Christos Chinopoulos:**

I believe in the metabolic approach to cancer therapy. Key to this approach is an understanding of the differences between the type of metabolism carried out by healthy cells, and the type of metabolism carried out by cancer cells. Once this is understood, cancer can be addressed from a metabolic point of view, which means cutting off the energy supply to the tumor.

Additionally, we know that cancer cells need certain metabolites, such as L-proline and arginine.[218] Healthy cells also require these metabolites, but not all at the same time, and they are less dependent upon them than cancer cells. This means that if we are able to very briefly block the provision of these metabolites to a tumor or to the vessels that supply a tumor, the tumor won't be able to survive.

The focus of my work is on identifying the metabolic pathways that are pertinent to tumor cells versus healthy cells. We believe that if we can identify the biological pathways that are used by a tumor but not used by healthy tissues, then we will know the primary pathways for chemotherapeutic intervention.

# Could the unique microbiome of tumors be used to diagnose or treat cancer?

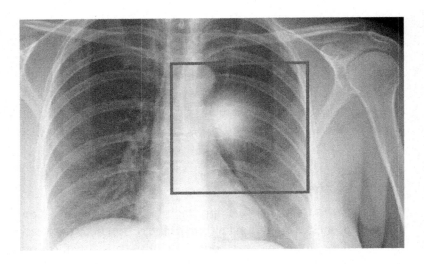

**Mahmoud Ghannoum:**

In our first study on the microbiome of tumors, we looked as metabolites in head and neck squamous cell carcinoma. By virtue of metabolomics and sequencing technology, we were able to characterize these metabolites, as well as compare them to the metabolites in normal cells.

To our amazement, we found that there are 22 different metabolites, eight of which were overproduced in the tumor tissue.[219] We dug a bit deeper and identified one particular chemical called 2-hydroxyglutarate (2-HG), which is present only in tumor tissues. This is very interesting, because it suggests to us that it is possible to use 2-HG as a biomarker of disease.[219]

In other words, detecting it in a patient's body would indicate that that patient has cancer. The beauty of this is that it can be detected noninvasively with the use of an oral wash—no need for painful surgical biopsies.[219] Larger clinical trials will be needed to validate these findings.

**Thomas Seyfried:**

Valaciclovir is an anti-viral medication that targets some of the microbes in the tumor microbiome, and it's been shown to slow the development of glioblastoma by a small amount.[220]

However, the bottom line is that cancer cells use glucose and glutamine no matter what.[25] This means that if glucose and glutamine are eliminated as fuel for the cancer cell, the cancer cell will die…and so too will the microbes. The goal is to get rid of the cancer, at which point the microbes become irrelevant.

**Carlo Maley:**

While there has been increased interest in the interaction between the microbiome and therapeutic response, the results are largely unknown. That said, I do think that the use of probiotics to increase a particular type of microbe could be therapeutically beneficial.

One of the issues on this topic is that gut microbes can affect the metabolism of cancer drugs.[221] For instance, prodrugs have to be metabolized in the liver by human cells before they actually become effective, but I would not be surprised if some of these drugs are actually being metabolized by the microbes. If so, then the types of microbes present in the gut would have a significant impact on the way therapy plays out.

**Richard White III:**

A recent paper published in *Microbiome* discusses the discovery of thousands of previously unknown phages in the human gut,[222] and we know that some phages confer protection to the host—potentially even against cancer. For example, phages have been shown to decrease the production of reactive oxygen species (ROS),[223] which damage DNA and promote tumor development and progression.[224]

Other phages have been shown to prevent alcohol-related liver disease in mice,[225] and reduce gastrointestinal inflammation.[226]

All of this contributes to an ongoing and exciting area of research.

**William Miller Jr.:**

Cancer cells are self-referential, smart, and creative problem solvers, and so are immune cells. This is an understanding that should shape our thinking when it comes to addressing the problem of cancer in new ways—ways that go beyond immunological lines. The problem of cancer is much more than just a biochemical phenomenon.

One way to address cancer is by manipulating the tumor microbiome by concentrating on concepts of co-engineering, co-partnering niche construction. One of the primary ways cells co-engineer is through stigmergic cues, which are small traces that every organism leaves in an environment after performing some sort of action. For example, when building mounds, termites and ants leave behind chemical signals that others can follow. Similarly, cells leave behind stigmergic cues.[227]

This is an entirely new level of cell-to-cell communication that I believe has not been deeply evaluated to date, and it's a very fertile, different way of looking at cancer dynamics. However, to manipulate a tumor microenvironment means to counter a skillful, selfish cancer cell. How can that be accomplished?

It may be possible by disrupting the cancer cell's ability to explore the environment. In other words, the goal is to deprive cancer cells of the resources they need. This is something that's certainly been worked on, but not necessarily from the point of view that cancer cells are intelligent problem solvers.

For instance, cancer cells have a unique ability to recruit other cells for assistance and can disguise themselves in such a way as to influence other cells to freely trade with them and get cheated in the process. Finding a way to block these abilities might be a good place to start.

# Emerging, novel approaches to cancer treatment

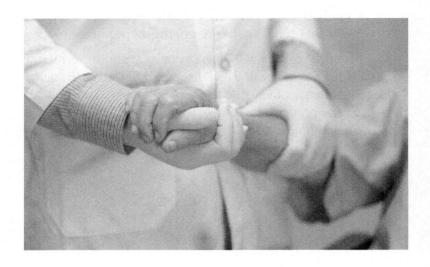

**Steven Eisenberg:**

"You have cancer."

Those three words can change a person's life and put them in an instantaneous post-traumatic or fight-or-flight state. For most people, those three words equate to "I'm going to die," and in a second, they are thrust into a world of tests, biopsies, and treatment options; a world of fear and uncertainty.

This is the human side of cancer, and it's the main reason I decided to become an oncologist. As an oncologist, it's my job to build upon the patient's hope, and to alleviate some of that fear and uncertainty during every single interaction.

It's also my job to deliver first-rate medical care, but to do so from the heart with empathy and compassion—just like I would if the patient were my own family.

Decades of research shows that patients who receive compassionate care have measurably better health outcomes than those who don't.[228-232] This is because with compassionate care, the patient's mind-body connection becomes an ally. The trifecta is good medicine, good mind, good body, and I don't think there is any field of medicine where this is more important than oncology.

The first thing I do with any patient is actually something I *don't* do: I don't bring a darn computer into the room. This is huge, because doctors, nurse practitioners, and physician assistants alike are drowning in the red tape of electronic medical records. Good records are important, of course, but don't bring the computer in the room and just stare at the screen. Instead, look into the eyes of the patient and have a scribe handle documentation. Oncologists cannot forget the importance of eye contact.

A physical exam can be done in a compassionate manner, or in a sterile manner. When I'm listening to a patient's heart, I'm speaking to the *patient* about what I'm saying, and the scribe is recording it. I'll place a hand on the patient's shoulder and say, "Good job, give me a deep breath," because a simple touch on the should is transformative. Doctors are forgetting these very simple things that make all the difference.

In oncology, we have the best technologies, like CAR T-Cell immunotherapy, biologics, and molecular genomics. But in my opinion, the better and better we get with the molecular technology, the further and further we get from the human being sitting right in front of us. That's a shame.

My book, *Love is the Strongest Medicine: Notes from a Cancer Doctor on Connection, Creativity, and Compassion,* aims to remind doctors about why they entered the profession of medicine in the first place. It's about bringing empathy and compassion to the human being that's suffering in front of them, because *not* doing this will not only hurt the patient, but the doctor as well. This is evidenced by the fact that one in two doctors is now experiencing severe symptoms of burnout.[233] They have a lack of empathy, they're just going through the motions, some are using alcohol and drugs to cope with the stress of being a doctor, and they're barely making it through each day.

Through the process of writing *Love is the Strongest Medicine*, I've learned so much about doctor burnout and its impact on patients. I've decided to start a mastermind group for doctors called Doctors Without Burnout. We will be supporting one another in video conferences every month, and creating a revolution in self-compassion so that doctors can refuel and avoid this horrible, progressive burnout that's happening in the world right now.

**Nathan Crane:**

"There is a cure for cancer; it's called your immune system," says Dr. Thomas Lodi in my documentary, Cancer: The Integrative Perspective. One of the core things we have to do is recognize that if someone has a fully functioning immune system, then they don't have to worry about getting cancer.

I believe millions of lives could be spared if medical schools started teaching about the impact of diet, lifestyle, environment, mindset, and emotions on the immune system, and how these factors can be the key to causing cancer, but also the key to preventing or reversing it.

I've talked to many medical doctors who have realized that surgery, radiation, chemotherapy, and other pharmaceuticals do not actually help their patients heal; they mask the symptoms of cancer rather than address the root cause of it. Focusing on the root cause led them to natural medicine, holistic medicine, and eventually integrative medicine.

Every single integrative medical doctor I've worked with has told me they see significantly better results in every single patient when using an integrative approach rather than a purely conventional approach to medicine. These doctors help their patients by focusing primarily on cutting-edge, non-toxic technologies, lifestyle changes, nutritional changes, mindset changes, and emotional healing.

The last two of these—mindset changes and emotional healing—are critical. Several case studies show that a person who is given a prognosis (e.g., six months to live) and believes it, focuses on it, and worries about it constantly will die exactly when it was predicted they would (if not from the disease, from something else).

Our beliefs are extremely powerful, and there's science to back it up. Bruce Lipton is one of the fathers of epigenetics and author of The Biology of Belief, in which he presents the science behind how our thoughts can literally create disease in the body, or help our bodies heal from disease.[234]

If a person doesn't believe they can heal and they don't have the strategies to heal, then they'll never heal; if a person doesn't believe they can heal but they do have the strategies to heal, then they may or may not heal. But if a person believes they can heal AND they have the strategies to do so, their odds of reversing cancer increase exponentially.

For the past ten years, it's been my mission to spread this information and make those strategies easily accessible. This is why I've created the Becoming Cancer-Free masterclass, which involves seven steps over nine modules, and covers everything that impacts people's internal and external environments.

From evidence-based nutritional medicine, to worksheets for removing every single toxin from the home, to medicinal movement and exercise, to meditation and positive beliefs and thinking patterns, this masterclass guides people through it all.

**Carlo Maley:**

I'm excited about applying evolutionary ideas to cancer therapy. These ideas stem primarily from agricultural practices and pest management, where the same problems exist: A field is sprayed with a pesticide that kills most pests, but also selects for mutant pests that are resistant to the pesticide. Similarly, a tumor is treated with chemotherapy that kills most of the cancer cells, but also selects for mutant cells that are resistant to the chemotherapy.

A variety of ideas has been developed in agriculture for dealing with and controlling pests. The key point here is that the goal is to control rather than eradicate pests. If the same strategy could be applied to the treatment of cancer, it would create radical change in the field of oncology. Just imagine cancer as a manageable chronic disease like diabetes, as opposed to an acutely lethal disease.

This strategy of controlling rather than eradicating is closely related to what's called evolutionary herding, which is the idea of using drugs to select for particular states in order to herd the population in a desirable direction.

Robert Gatenby came up with something called double bind therapy, which is based on the idea of using one drug to select for tumor cells that will be vulnerable to a second drug.[235] I developed a similar strategy called the "sucker's gambit," which is based on the idea of using one drug to eliminate the tumor cells that will be resistant to the second (main) drug.[236] While these strategies haven't been developed fully, they've generated a lot of interest.

Another exciting idea that has come out of the agricultural and pest management field is called adaptive therapy, which is based on the fitness cost of resistance. To elaborate, some resistant cells have a mechanism for pumping out chemicals before those chemicals can kill them. However, these pumps consume about half of all of the energy budget of the cell, so there is a big cost. If there aren't any chemicals that need to be pumped out, the resistant cells pay a huge cost for no benefit.

This means that in the absence of drugs, resistant cells have a disadvantage against sensitive cells, which also means that with the careful application of drugs, sensitive cells can be maintained and used as a way to keep resistant cells under control for longer periods of time.

This strategy does not depend on a particular drug nor a particular type of cancer. Further, it doesn't require FDA approval of a new drug; it only requires clinical trials demonstrating that these strategies (i.e., maintaining sensitive cells and controlling cancer on a long-term basis) lead to longer survival times and better quality of life than the standard care.

One human clinical trial has already demonstrated just that,[237] and more trials are set to begin soon.

**Ruchi Gaba:**

Something very new on the horizon is radiofrequency ablation (RFA), a procedure whereby a needle electrode is inserted into cancerous tissue, and high-frequency energy passes through the needle to destroy cancer cells.

RFA has been around since 2006 and is often used in some countries, including Italy and Korea, but it is just starting to be adopted in the U.S. Currently, most uses of RFA are on benign tumors or nodules, but data from the U.S. about its use in cancer will be coming soon.

**Anonymous:**

Traditionally, radiation has been given in very small doses, typically on a schedule of Monday through Friday over the course of six to eight weeks. Small doses are used in order to allow normal tissues time to recover from the associated DNA damage.

Stereotactic body radiation therapy (SBRT) is a new technology that decreases radiation damage to normal tissues[238] by implanting radioactive seeds and bypassing normal tissues that surround cancerous tissues.

Traditional radiotherapy for left-sided breast cancer results in the radiation field passing directly through the heart. Stereotactic body radiation therapy avoids this by delivering radiotherapy when the patient takes a deep breath in, causing the chest wall to pull away from the heart. There are also techniques that allow for very high doses of radiation to be delivered to small and specific areas while sparing the normal surrounding tissue.

Most breast cancer patients can finish this treatment within one to three weeks,[238] which is generating the latest and greatest excitement in the radiation field.

Meanwhile, there is a lot of preclinical research being conducted on ways to alter metabolism in order to improve the efficacy of radiation. This research is still in the Petri dish stage, but could hold great promise.

**Kimberly Bussey:**

If the atavistic theory of cancer is true, then cancer has reverted to a reliance upon essential unicellular processes, and these processes could be therapeutically targeted. However, we have to remember that applying any type of therapy to an organism is like asking that organism (or associated phenotype) to adapt in such a way as to avoid that therapy.

For this reason, it's important to apply therapies wisely, so that cancers adapt in such a way as to become more communal and cooperative, and to return toward multicellularity. When cancers do this, their growth slows or ceases altogether. The idea is to steer tumor evolution toward multicellular processes and away from unicellular processes.

**François Fuks:**

The epigenetic discoveries that we are making are clearly changing the way we can diagnose and treat cancer. Epigenetic therapy for cancer is already a reality, and some FDA-approved drugs for DNA methylation are currently being used. However, these drugs have many side effects as a result of inhibiting DNA methylation on every given gene (including normal genes) as opposed to specific cancer genes.

These drugs might well be called epigenetic drugs of the first generation; next will be second-generation epigenetic drugs that confer the benefits of greater specificity, such as fewer side effects. Research on this front is ongoing, and there are currently over 30 epigenetic drugs being tested in clinical trials.

In the coming years, some of these drugs will be used more broadly in patients and hopefully in many different types of cancer. This is a very active and exciting area in oncology.


**Mustafa Djamgoz:**

One of the remarkable properties of the sodium channel in metastasis is that it is embryonic; it is expressed in its neonatal splice form.[239]

To elaborate, we are all born with approximately 22,000 genes. As neonates, these genes are organized in a certain way. Imagine that these genes are like beads on a string, strung or organized in such a way as to subserve neonatal needs. Once we are born and begin developing, these 22,000 genes get restrung or reorganized in such a way as to subserve the needs of the adult body.

This relates to cancer because many of the genes in tumor cells undergo dedifferentiation, a process by which they revert to an earlier state—the embryonic state. The more dedifferentiated a tumor, the more embryonic it is and the more aggressive it is, but no one knows why. My guess is that something in the body detects the presence of cancerous tissue and/or the resultant disruption in organ function, and attempts to fix it by rebuilding and editing the tissues, which requires the genes to return to the embryonic form.

The same thing seems to happen with the sodium channel: In tumor cells (including micrometastases), the sodium channel is in the embryonic form, but in other cells, the sodium channel is in the adult form. To make these channels clinically useful, we used molecular biology to identify the differences between the embryonic and adult forms of the channel. Based on those differences, we recently succeeded in making a monoclonal antibody that recognizes only the embryonic form of the channel, which sits only on tumor cells.[240] The embryonic and adult forms of the sodium channel are also distinguishable pharmacologically thus raising the possibility of developing cancer-specific small-molecule drugs (SMDs).[260]

The idea is to deliver this monoclonal antibody (or SMD) into the circulation, where it will travel around the body and bind only to tumor cells, including those in micro-metastatic sites. To destroy micro-metastases, all we need to do is attach a cytotoxic agent to the antibody; the antibody will target the cancer cells, and the cytotoxic agent will kill them.

If we can manage this, it will be a tremendous achievement.

Yet another approach to treatment stems from our finding that under the hypoxic conditions of a tumor, voltage-gated sodium channels stay open for far longer than they do under normal conditions in normal cells.[105] This causes a huge influx of sodium into cancer tissues, which leads to proteolysis and eventually metastasis (see my answer to question #16).

It is hypoxia that causes the sodium channel to remain open. This happens not only in tumors, but any place in the body where oxygen levels are insufficient. For example, this happens in the heart during arrhythmia, angina, and cardiac arrest.

This led us to consider repurposing an antianginal drug used in cardiology. We have patented this drug on the basis of secondary medical use. It has already been tested on animals, where it has shown to work very well in both breast and prostate cancer.[241] Since it is a well-known drug with an established safety profile, we can bypass toxicity tests and move it into the clinic.

The field of oncology has been flabbergasted by this kind of research, if for no reason other than the significant involvement of ion channels and electrical signals in tumors. The field of cancer bioelectricity (sometimes also called 'cancer neuroscience') is becoming well accepted and buzzing with activity all over the world and offering real clinical potential.

**Michael Levin**:

Given sufficient resources, I believe bioelectricity could become the basis of biomedical products for diagnosing and treating cancer. It's not unreasonable to say that this will happen within the next five years, but I certainly don't want to predict an exact timeline.

I believe there will be improved diagnostics with the use of voltage-sensitive dyes that allow for the detection of precancerous tissues, and there might even be a topical cream that can be applied to the skin and oral mucosa that makes electrically-aberrant cells visible.

On the treatment side of things, I predict that surgeons will be using voltage-sensitive dyes to visualize tumor margins during resection procedures, which will allow for certainty when it comes to the question of whether an entire tumor has been removed.

I also think computational modeling will be used to analyze a particular patient's physiology and genetics to come up with the ideal blend of ion channel drugs designed to normalize the electrical state of specific tissues. I am optimistic about this normalization strategy, especially since it will be a hell of a lot better than chemotherapy.

# CO-AUTHOR BIOS

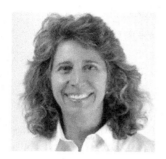

> **SANDY BEVACQUA**
> Email: wish2@wish4life.com

Dr. Sandy holds a PhD. in Molecular and Cellular Biology. She has worked as a research scientist in both university and government settings and has lectured to the public and to medical professionals around the globe since 1986.

With her background in the fields of genetic engineering and human tumor biology, Dr. Sandy makes the complex interactions between our bodies, the foods we eat, supplements we take and lifestyles we lead, understandable and memorable.

Implementing her expertise in Blood Biochemistry and Molecular Genetics, Dr. Sandy is able to offer guidance (backed by peer-reviewed scientific research) to achieve the biochemical balance that research tells us we all require to experience optimal health and vitality. By understanding your unique biochemistry and genetics, you can discover valuable information about your body and its distinctive needs. You become an empowered advocate for your own health!

Personal one-on-one sessions are available as well as Educational Online Courses, E-Books, and MP4 downloads at www.DrSandyBevacqua.com

Dr Sandy is also available as your medical advocate. She can provide your analysis and pertinent research to your healthcare provider to help you get the best care possible.

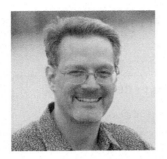

**PERRY MARSHALL**

Email: perry@perrymarshall.com

Perry Marshall is one of the most expensive business strategists in the world. He is endorsed in FORBES and INC Magazine and has authored eight books. At London's Royal Society he announced the world's largest science research challenge, the $10 million Evolution 2.0 Prize.

His reinvention of the Pareto Principle is published in Harvard Business Review, and his Google book laid the foundations for the $100 billion Pay Per Click industry. He has a degree in Engineering and lives with his family in Chicago.

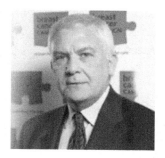

**MUSTAFA DJAMGOZ**
Email: m.djamgoz@imperial.ac.uk

Following my physics degree education at Imperial College London, I fulfilled my childhood dream of studying the body's electricity, initially (and for 25 years) on the electrophysiology of retinal neurones but also on a variety of other model neural systems. The whole of my academic career has been spent at Imperial, rising to Professor of Neurobiology in 1995. Curiosity took me to studying electrical signalling in cancer cells where I discovered the voltage-gated sodium channel as an engine of cancer progression. In 2005, this led to my second personal chair as Professor of Cancer Biology. In 2021, I retired from active academia and was appointed Emeritus Professor at Imperial. I now spend most of my professional time further advancing the new field of cancer research I call 'neuroscience solutions to cancer'! This is aimed at developing non-toxic drugs to enable 'living with cancer' chronically!

The behaviour of living cells is influenced by both their genetics and by their environment. In this module, you will explore how the genetic information in cells is expressed as a phenotype, and how this expression is regulated in response to stimuli from the cell's environment. The module will address the central information transfer pathways in the cell (replication, transcription and translation), and aims to develop your skills in analysing genetic systems in model organisms. It will familiarise you with the compartments from which eukaryotic cells are constructed and how proteins are targeted to them. We will also explore specific examples of cellular interactions: neuronal signalling, vertebrate immunity, and viral infection.

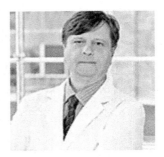

**LÁSZLÓ BOROS**

I am currently the chief scientist of SIDMAP and the Deutenomics Science Institute and a former Professor of Pediatrics at the University of California Los Angeles (UCLA) School of Medicine. I also co-directed the Stable Isotope Research Laboratory at the Lundquist Institute for Biomedical Innovations (LUNDQUIST) and participated as an investigator at the Clinical and Translational Research Institute at the Harbor-UCLA Medical Center with a primary focus on studying cancer cell metabolism with the use of a specifically designed 13C-glucose tracer and mass spectroscopy.

Born and educated in Hungary, my medical background includes three years of gastroenterology and pancreatology, focusing on chronic pancreatitis and pancreatic cancer. I spent two years as a visiting scholar in Essen, Germany, studying various animal models of chronic pancreatitis.

In 1990, I moved to Columbus, Ohio, and joined the history-making laboratory of Drs. Zollinger and Ellison, who discovered hormonal regulatory mechanisms involved in pancreatic cancer growth where I trained in biochemistry, diagnostics and integrative treatments.

In 1995 I became the lead investigator to clinically apply 13C and 2H (deuterium) based stable isotope technologies to study diabetes and cancer cell growth in vitro, in animal models and human cohorts at UCLA.

I am an expert in using metabolic profiling and mitochondrial nanomechanics to the further understanding of particularly aggressive cancers. I also participate in research projects targeting population metabolic disorders, such as diabetes and obesity, and I am involved in discovering the underlying mechanisms of rare metabolic disorders arising from genetic mutations affecting vitamin transport.

I am an internationally recognized expert of metabolic water biochemistry as well as deuterium mediated kinetic isotopic effects in health and disease, which are translational fields of Deutenomics in medicine. My most recent studies target deupletion and deuposition related mechanisms as the result of intra-cellular hydrophobic lipid membrane nanoconfinements via the quantum destabilization and delocalization of protons in metabolic water.

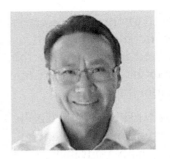

**ERIC FUNG**

Email: efung@grailbio.com

Executive with experience in IVD test development (including biomarker discovery, validation, clinical trials, FDA submission, product launch). Successful tests include OVA1, the first FDA cleared multivariate protein IVD assay blood test for ovarian cancer; Athena clinical trial for HPV test; and CytoScan Dx Assay, the first genome-wide copy number cytogenetics assay (chromosomal microarray). Successful in large, medium, and small companies and comfortable with all key stakeholders: colleagues across all departments, customers, investors, FDA, KOLs.

Participated in three successful financing rounds ($21MM and $43MM PIPE's, $21MM Follow-on). >55 publications and 14 issued patents.

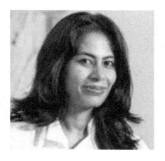

**JYOTSNA BATRA**

Email: jyotsna.batra@qut.edu.au

Dr Jyotsna Batra is an Advance Queensland Industry Research Fellow at the Australian Prostate Cancer Research Centre-Queensland, QUT, Australia. She has studied Biochemistry towards a Master's degree and obtained her PhD in Biotechnology working on the genetic complexity of the heredity disorders.

Associate Professor Jyotsna Batra is leading a research group on molecular genetics of prostate cancer. Her current research focus is to identify cancer risk-associated genetic variants and to understand their molecular consequences on cancer initiation and progression. She aims to develop better biomarker to detect cancer early and to identify genetic biomarkers which can distinguish slow growing disease from very aggressive prostate cancer at an early stage, so that better decision on therapeutic interventions can be made.

Dr Batra has contributed to >100 research articles, including that in high impact journals such as Cancer Discovery and Nature Genetics. Dr Batra has received several poster and oral prizes for her research work (N=42). She has been a finalist for the prestigious ASMR Postdoctoral Award and Women in Technology (WiT) Rising Star Award and has been awarded QUT VC Excellence Award (2015) and Performance Award (2016) and Cure Cancer Researcher of the Year (2018).

She has attracted >11M in funding and is currently funded by NHMRC, Cancer Council Queensland and Can TOO, Cure Cancer and Cancer Australia Foundation Young Investigator grants and DoD Idea Development projects.

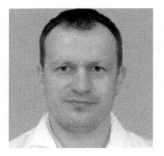

**ANDRIY MARUSYK**

Email: Andriy.Marusyk@moffitt.org

The main focus of research in my lab is understanding of how cancers adapt to therapies. This entail understanding both intrinsic changes that happen within tumor cells, as well as extrinsic impact of tumor microenvironments. For example, paracrine factors produced by non-malignant cells within tumors (such as fibroblasts), can greatly blunt sensitivity of cancer cells to therapies, enabling some tumor cells to survive, but also reducing drug-induced selection pressures. The ultimate goal is to use this knowledge to develop therapies that optimize long term outcomes by combining suppression of tumor growth with hindering their ability to develop resistance.

Tumors can be viewed as complex eco-systems, where evolving populations of genetically and phenotypically heterogeneous malignant cells are engaged in a network of reciprocal interactions with multiple normal cell types and non-cellular components of tumor micro and macro environment. Mainstream reductionistic molecular oncology studies have revealed molecular mechanisms responsible for malignant phenotypes (aka "hallmarks of cancers") in great mechanistic detail, enabling the development of highly effective targeting therapies. Unfortunately, these therapies are rarely curative, as, owing to microenvironmental complexity and tumor heterogeneity they fail to eliminate all of the tumor cells, allowing cancers to evolve adaptations to therapy induced selective pressures, ultimately resulting in relapsed disease. Thus, despite the spectacular developments in understanding proximal mechanisms of the disease, this knowledge has not yet resulted in dramatic improvements of clinical outcomes.

We believe that in order to break the impasse, we need to account for tumor complexity, which can be achieved by combining knowledge of proximal mechanisms with an eco-evolutionary framework to understand how tumors change in space and time. - The Marusyk Lab/ MOffitt Cancer Center

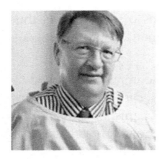

**BRENDON COVENTRY**

Email:
brendon.coventry@adelaide.edu.au

Brendon Coventry BMBS PhD FRACS FACS FRSM is a surgical oncologist, immunologist, and medical researcher from Adelaide, South Australia. He is an Associate Professor of Surgery at The University of Adelaide, Fellow of the Royal Australasian College of Surgeons, American College of Surgeons, & Royal Society of Medicine, and holds a PhD in Immunology & Cancer Immunotherapy. Coventry's research contributions have been made in the field of Immunology, Surgery & Public Health. In 2014, he published a seven-volume series widely used on Risks & Complications in Surgery with Springer Publishing, selling over 70,000 copies. He has been a NIH Chief Investigator of the Sentinel Lymph Node trials with Dr Donald Morton, proving the technique of Selective Sentinel Node Dissection for improving Melanoma Surgery with several publications in the New England Journal of Surgery.

**Melanoma Vaccine**

Beginning in the late 1990s, Coventry noticed that some of his patients with advanced melanoma, unable to be removed using surgery, responded very well to melanoma vaccines causing all of their melanoma to disappear. Since then, some patients have survived more than 20-years. Other patients, despite receiving identical treatment, were not cured. Coventry was able to increase complete response rates to treatment of advanced melanoma from <1% with standard chemotherapy to 17% with vaccines, and without significant negative side effects. Observations led him to speculate that the immune system operates in a cyclical manner, with peaks and troughs - evidenced by measurable fluctuations in serum biomarkers such as C-reactive protein (CRP), indicating an immune biorhythm.

Publishing in the Journal of Translational Medicine in 2009, Coventry led a team which demonstrated that the immune cycle could be seen in fluctuating levels of C-reactive protein in the blood of a given patient. According to Coventry, "[t]he immune system works in waves that seems to be switching on and off constantly. And now what we're trying to do is see whether we can identify periods or phases in that cycle where we could target the vaccine more effectively..."Crucially, the ability to administer treatment at the most effective time in a patient's immune cycle means that significantly smaller dosages of chemotherapy can be used, which in turn means far fewer negative side effects to treatment.

Coventry, in his capacity as Research Director of the Australian Melanoma Research Foundation, has appeared before committees of the Parliament of Australia. In a 2014 submission to the Standing Committee on Health into Skin Cancer in Australia, it was stated that without the application of the new knowledge on the immune cycle cancer treatment was a "mathematically random" process. The 2015 submission to the Senate Standing Committee on Community Affairs Inquiry into the Availability of new, innovative and specialist cancer drugs in Australia states that the five-year survival rate of patients with advanced cancer is consistent with statistical probability that a patient's treatment will be administered at exactly the right place in their immune cycle.

Operating on this theory, further research has shown that the oscillations in the immune biorhythms are complex, partially disproving the initial idea of strictly regular cycles based on the initial fundamental mathematics. By defining an artificial intelligence approach with Dr Dorraki & Prof Abbott the way for more accurate therapeutic applications using complex mathematical analysis and new machine learning approaches has been designed.

Recent work has proposed 'vaccination' as the central mechanism for probably all cancer therapies, likely with evolutionary origins, leading to new possibilities for vaccine therapeutic design for effective cancer treatments.

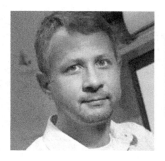

**GÁBOR BALÁZSI**
Email: gabor.balazsi@stonybrook.edu

Gábor Balázsi received his undergraduate Physics degree at the Babeş-Bolyai University in Cluj/Kolozsvár, Romania. In 2001 he completed a Physics PhD in noise-induced cell dynamics at the University of Missouri at Saint Louis. From 2002 - 2005, as a Systems Biology postdoctoral fellow at Northwestern University, he studied gene-regulatory network response to environmental perturbations.

From 2005 - 2006, as a Synthetic Biology postdoctoral fellow at the Center for Biodynamics of Boston University he developed synthetic gene circuits to study how cellular diversity promotes drug resistance. As Assistant Professor at the University of Texas MD Anderson Cancer Center, from 2006 – 2014 he built a growing library of synthetic gene control circuits in yeast and human cells. He was among the recipients of the 2009 NIH Director's New Innovator Award, which aims to "stimulate highly innovative research and support promising new investigators".

Since 2014, as the Henry Laufer Professor of Physical and Quantitative Biology at Stony Brook University, his interdisciplinary research team has been developing and evolving synthetic gene circuits to understand drug resistance and cancer progression. His research group is part-experimental and part-computational, fostering interdisciplinary training while advancing the frontiers of quantitative biology.

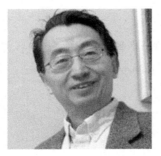

**HENRY HENG**

Email: hheng@med.wayne.edu

Our group is searching for a new framework of cancer/organismal evolution and its clinical implications. On the theoretical level, we have introduced the Genome Architecture Theory that considers genomic topology (or karyotype) as a new layer of key genetic information, and the genome defined "system inheritance" rather than gene/epi-gene defined "parts inheritance" represents the blueprint of bio-system.

From our experimental work, we have discovered "two phases of cancer evolution" (punctuated macro-cellular evolution and stepwise Darwinian micro-cellular evolution) that are commonly detected during the entire process of cancer formation (including immortalization, transformation, metastasis to drug resistance). Within the punctuated phase, the genome chaos dominates, which explains the rapid cancer evolution beyond individual cancer genes.

We have also established the concept/methodology of measuring genome instability based on the frequency of non-clonal chromosome aberrations, which is essential to understand the diverse molecular mechanisms of cancer in the context of somatic cell evolution.

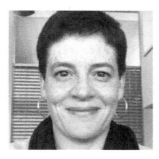

**KIMBERLY BUSSEY, PH.D.**
Email: kbusse@midwestern.edu

Dr. Bussey is a cancer cytogeneticist, applied bioinformatician, and an assistant professor in the Precision Medicine Program at Midwestern University. She is passionate about educating healthcare professionals about genomics and how to integrate genomics into their current medical decision making. Her research centers around understanding how large-scale chromosome alterations in tumors lead to cancer. Her motivation, the observation that cancer is an evolutionary process characterized by chromosome evolution, has led her to interdisciplinary collaborations with engineers, theoretical physicists, and artists to study both common and rare cancers in academic, government, non-profit, and industry settings.

An alumna of the University of Arizona, Dr. Bussey received her PhD in Medical and Molecular Genetics from Oregon Health and Science University in 2000 and completed a post-doctoral fellowship in bioinformatics at the National Cancer Institute. She has published 40+ scientific papers and has been granted six patents for her work, with an additional patent application pending. She is actively involved with Interface: Faith and Science at Pinnacle, a forum for the exploration of science, faith, and their intersection in modern life. When she isn't doing science, Dr. Bussey enjoys playing music (piano and English hand bells), hiking, mountain biking, and indulging in her passion for Star Wars with her husband and two daughters.

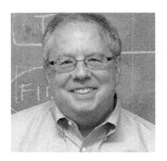

**ROBERT GATENBY**

Email: robert.gatenby@moffitt.org,
geraldine.rodriguez@moffitt.org

Clinical oncology investigations have largely focused on new drug discovery. Since Ehrlich's pioneering work more than a century ago, his concept of a "magic bullet," a drug that can kill cancer cells while sparing normal host cells, has dominated the ongoing quest for a cure for cancer. In the vast global drug development industry that has emerged from this concept, the focus is almost entirely on identifying new and better drugs. This approach has worked very well in developing many novel and successful agents for cancer therapy.

However, most metastatic cancers remain fatal because even highly effective treatments usually fail due to evolution of resistance. Arguably, Darwinian dynamics are thus the proximate cause of death in many cancer patients.

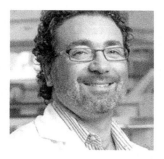

**SAVERIO GENTILE**

Email: sgentile@uic.edu

Dr. Saverio Gentile is an Assistant Professor in the Departments of Hematology and Oncology at the University of Illinois College of Medicine. As a postdoctoral fellow at the National Institute of Environmental Health Sciences (NIEHS/NIH) and later in the Cardiology Department at Duke University, he carried out a multi-approach investigation on the role of voltage-gated potassium and calcium channels activity in epithelial derivative cells including cancer cells and neurons. He has a strong background in electrophysiology, calcium imaging, biochemistry, molecular biology, cell biology and signal transduction.

Dr. Gentile developed a successful technical approach that allowed dissecting ion channels-dependent activation of biochemical pathways in cancer. He demonstrated a record of successful and productive research projects in an area of high relevance for ion channel dependent diseases. Dr. Gentile successfully collaborated with other researchers in different fields and produced several peer-reviewed publications. Dr. Gentile is the scientist behind a recently activated clinical trial in which the anticancer effects of a potassium channel activator molecule will be tested on ovarian cancer patients.

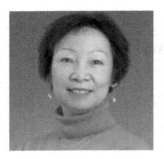

**LI ZHANG**

Email: li.zhang@uhnresearch.ca

Dr. Li Zhang obtained her M.D. from Anhui Medical University, in China and Ph.D. from the Leiden University in the Netherlands. She joined the faculty of Medicine at the University of Toronto in 1994 and is a Professor in the Departments of Laboratory Medicine and Pathobiology and Immunology at the University of Toronto. She holds a Maria H. Bacardi Chair in Transplantation.

Professor Zhang's research, supported by the Canadian Institutes of Health Research, Canadian Cancer Society Research Institute, the US Leukemia & Lymphoma Society and National Institutes of Health, has been focused on understanding the cellular and molecular mechanisms involved in immunity and tolerance and its applications in various diseases, including graft rejection, graft versus host disease and cancer.

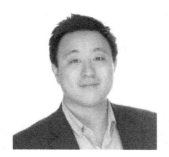

**JONG BOK LEE**

Email:
jongbok.lee@mail.utoronto.ca

Dr. Jong Bok Lee received his HBSc and Ph.D degree at the University of Toronto. He is an author of 12 peer-reviewed articles related to T cell biology. He is a recipient of several national awards including CIHR-Vanier scholarship.

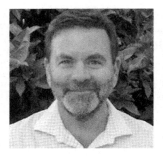

**GARY FORESMAN**

Email:
miranda@middlepathmedicine.com

Dr. Foresman is the only Internist on the Central Coast with extensive research training during medical school as part of the Junior Honors Medical Program. He ranked among the top in the nation on his Internal Medicine Board Exams. He has the best and most comprehensive Internal Medicine training to be found, including serving as a Clinical Professor who has trained other physicians at a University Medical Center.

In 1994, when he moved to the Central Coast to raise his family and open a private practice, he quickly became dissatisfied with the inability of established Western medical treatments to effectively treat many of his patients. Determined to help his patients, he began investigating alternative therapies and has expanded his training in many systems of healing, not just Ayurveda, Meditation, Stress Management, and Massage but also Botanical, Ortho Molecular and Functional Medicine Systems. Middle Path Medicine was founded in 2008 as Dr. Foresman continued to expand his knowledge base. His precise, scientific mind combined with a holistic integrative perspective makes him not only the best diagnostician, but also the most skilled at therapeutically synthesizing the finest healing modalities for each individual.

Middle Path Medicine's founder and President Gary E. Foresman, MD has over 25 years of experience in the clinical practice of Internal and Integrative Medicine. Read about his approach to medicine as well as his biography & certifications on Dr. Foresman's webpage. https://middlepathmedicine.com/

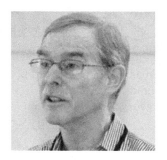

**JAMES SHAPIRO**

Email: jsha@uchicago.edu

James A. Shapiro has worked as professor of microbiology at the University of Chicago since 1973. Earlier, as a PhD student at Cambridge University in 1967, he was the first to recognize DNA transposons (is elements) in bacteria, and while working at Harvard Medical School in 1968, Shapiro headed the first team to isolate a single gene from a living organism. In 1976, he and two colleagues organized the first international meeting on mobile genetic elements, and in 1979 he published the first detailed molecular model of DNA transposition.

An expert in bacterial genetics, he proposes the concept of natural genetic engineering, which encompasses an array of biochemical functions that account for novel DNA structures created in the process of biological evolution. Shapiro is an advocate of non-Darwinian evolution and is a critic of the modern synthesis. He has published primary scientific literature on evolution since the early 90s. Early this year (2022), he is publishing a 2nd edition of his book Evolution: A View from the 21st Century. Fortified.

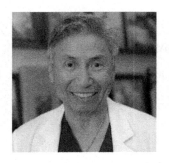

**GEORGE YU**

Email: clinical georgewyumd@gmail.com and professional george.yu8@gmail.com

George W. Yu was trained in general surgery at the Peter Bent Brigham Harvard Medical Center and Johns Hopkins in his subspecialty urological and pelvic oncology and reconstruction. In addition, he has had a wide experience as a missionary surgeon working with great surgeon such as Doctor Irvin and Dennis Burkitt in Africa.

He has been clinical professor of Urology at the George Washington University Medical Center and partner in Aegis Medical and Research Associates for the last 35 thirty-five years in Washington DC and Annapolis Maryland.

Since 2006, the YuFoundation.org was created by his generous patrons with focuses on nutritional mitochondrial metabolism, sex hormones in health aging and disease, cell regeneration and stem cell research and methods of removal of toxic chemical from our bodies.

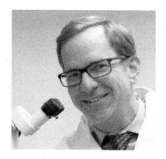

**BEN STANGER**
Email: bstanger@upenn.edu

Ben Stanger, MD PhD is Hanna Wise Professor in Cancer Research at the University of Pennsylvania, where he has studied gastrointestinal cancer for the past 15 years.

**Pancreas Cancer**

Pancreatic Ductal Adenocarcinoma (PDA) is poised to become the second leading cause of cancer death in the United States. This poor outcome is attributable to two facts:

(1) pancreatic cancers metastasize early, before clinical detection, and
(2) current anti-cancer therapies are inadequate. Our laboratory tackles these problems by understanding how tumors metastasize and identifying vulnerabilities that will lead to better therapies. Our efforts include studies of the tumor immune microenvironment, tumor metabolism, and cellular plasticity and metastasis biology. We rely on genetically engineered mice that recapitulate salient features of the human disease, functional genomics, and in vitro culture methods that recapitulate the unique microenvironment of the tumor. In addition, we maintain a strong interest in liver biology and the pathogenesis of type I diabetes.

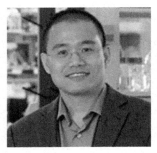

**YIBIN KANG**

Yibin Kang is a Warner-Lambert/Parke-Davis Professor of Molecular Biology at Princeton University and an Associate Director of Rutgers Cancer Institute of New Jersey. He is also a founder member of the Ludwig Institute for Cancer Research Princeton Branch. Dr. Kang graduated with a bachelor's degree from Fudan University in Shanghai in 1995. After completing his graduate study at Duke in 2000 and postdoctoral training with Dr. Joan Massagué at the Memorial Sloan-Kettering Cancer Center, he joined the faculty of Princeton University as an Assistant Professor of Molecular Biology in 2004. He was promoted to Associate Professor with tenure in 2010 and to Endowed Chair Full Professor in 2012. Dr. Kang has served as the President of the Metastasis Research Society (2016-2018) and Chair of the American Association for Cancer Research (AACR) Tumor Microenvironment Working Group (2018-2019).

Dr. Kang's research focuses on the molecular mechanisms of breast cancer metastasis. He has published over 180 research articles in leading journals including Science, Cancer Cell, and Nature Medicine. Dr. Kang's outstanding achievements have been recognized by many prestigious awards, including the 2011 Vicek Prize for Creative Promise in Biomedical Sciences, and the American Association for Cancer Research (AACR) Award for Outstanding Achievements in Cancer Research (2012), and the AACR Outstanding Investigator Award in Breast Cancer Research (2014). Dr. Kang was elected as a Fellow of

American Association for the Advancement of Science (AAAS) and a Komen Scholar in 2016 and an American Cancer Society Research Professor in 2019.

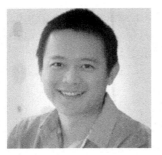

**XI HUANG**

Email: xi.huang@sickkids.ca

We study physical properties and mechano-electrical-chemical signaling in cancer. While extensive research has informed genetics and biochemical mechanisms in tumorigenesis, how mechanical and electrical signaling regulate cancer is less defined. Ion channels govern cell behaviors by perceiving physicochemical cues (mechanical force, membrane voltage, temperature, pH etc.) to control ion flux across membranes. We ask the following questions:

At the systematic level, what are the mutational landscape and functional alterations of ion channels in cancer?

At the tissue level, how do ion channels regulate tumor initiation, progression, metastasis, and drug resistance in genetically tractable animal models?

At the cellular level, how do ion channels perceive physicochemical cues to control cancer cell state?

At the molecular level, how do different ion channels form a functional network to regulate cancer cell behaviors?

Can we use ion channel-targeting drugs to treat cancer?

Using multi-disciplinary approaches in bioinformatics, Drosophila and mouse genetics, xenograft modeling, advanced imaging, electrophysiology, and bioengineering, we discover disease mechanisms and therapeutic vulnerabilities at the interface of cancer biology, neuroscience, and mechanobiology.

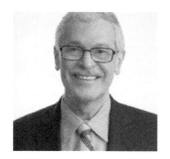

**MAHMOUD GHANNOUM**

Email: mag3@case.edu

My lab investigates fungal pathogens including Candida, Aspergillus and Cryptococcus, in addition to fungal virulence factors including phospholipase B, germination, adhesion, and biofilm formation. Dr. Ghannoum's research is focused on defining the role of the bacteriome and mycobiome (the bacterial and fungal community) in cancer and other health conditions. His expertise in the area of polymicrobial biofilms provides an important area of cancer research in view of the recent association of polymicrobial biofilms in colorectal cancer and Crohn's disease.

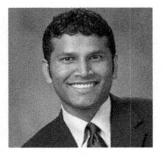

**SENDURAI MANI**

Email: mani@mdanderson.org

Sendurai A. Mani is a Professor in the Department of Translational Molecular Pathology at MD Anderson Cancer Center. He is also the co-director of the Metastasis Research Center and the Center for Stem Cell and Developmental Biology at MD Anderson Cancer Center. Dr. Mani was the first to demonstrate that cancer cells can become cancer stem cells by activating the embryonic epithelial-mesenchymal transition (EMT) program. This finding provided the foundation and explanation for the presence of plasticity within the tumor and the development of metastasis and resistance to treatments.

Dr. Mani has received numerous prizes and awards, including a V-Scholar Award, The American Cancer Society Research Scholar award, being elected as a full member of Sigma Xi, a scientific research honor society, and a fellow of the American Association for the Advancement of Sciences (AAAS).

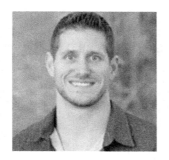

**NATHAN CRANE**
Email: nathancrane@me.com

Nathan Crane is an award-winning author, inspirational speaker, plant-based athlete, event producer and 20x award-winning documentary filmmaker. Nathan is the Founder of The Panacea Community, Creator of the Global Cancer Symposium, Host of the Conquering Cancer Summit, and Director and Producer of the documentary film, Cancer; The Integrative Perspective.

Nathan has received numerous awards for his contribution to health, healing, and personal development including the Accolade Film Competition 2020 Outstanding Achievement Humanitarian Award and the Outstanding Community Service Award from the California Senate for his work in education and empowerment with natural and integrative methods for healing cancer. With more than 15 years in the health and wellness field, Nathan has reached millions of people around the world with his inspiring messages of hope, healing and transformation.

Learn more at www.NathanCrane.com

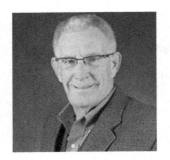

**THOMAS SEYFRIED**

Email: thomas.seyfried@bc.edu

Our research program focuses on mechanisms by which metabolic therapy manages chronic diseases such as epilepsy, neurodegenerative lipid storage diseases, and cancer. The metabolic therapies include caloric restriction, fasting, and ketogenic diets. Our approach is based on the idea that compensatory metabolic pathways are capable of modifying the pathogenesis of complex diseases.

Global shifts in metabolic environment can neutralize molecular pathology. In the case of cancer, these therapies target and kill tumor cells while enhancing the physiological health of normal cells. The neurochemical and genetic mechanisms of these phenomena are under investigation in novel animal models and include the processes of inflammation, cellular physiology, angiogenesis, and lipid biochemistry.

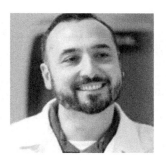

**CHRISTOS CHINOPOULOS**

Email:
chinopoulos.christos@med.semmelweis-univ.hu

Dr. Christos Chinopoulos' main research interest is oncometabolism, a topic that concerns the changes in the expression of proteins, mostly enzymes, 'rewiring' certain metabolic pathways. These alterations provide an excellent opportunity for cancer-specific therapeutic intervention.

Identifying those proteins involved in bioenergetic pathways that are up- or downregulated in order to serve the needs of neoplasia, is crucial for beating cancer. The RPPA facility of the Semmelweis University (http://rppa.hu) aims to quantify the expression of all mitochondrial proteins in healthy and solid tumor samples.

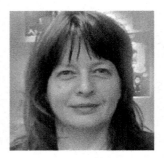

**KORNELIA POLYAK**

Email:
kornelia_polyak@dfci.harvard.edu

Our goal is to identify differences between normal and cancerous breast tissue, determine their consequences, and use this information to improve the clinical management of breast cancer patients. The three main areas of our interests are:

(1) how to accurately predict breast cancer risk and prevent breast cancer initiation or progression from in situ to invasive disease,

(2) better understand drivers of tumor evolution with special emphasis on metastatic progression and therapeutic resistance, and

(3) novel therapeutic targets in breast cancer with particular focus on aggressive cancers such as triple negative breast cancer and inflammatory breast cancer. All of our studies start with analyzing samples from breast cancer patients (or normal healthy women for the risk studies), formulate hypotheses based on our observations, use experimental models to test these, and then translate back our findings into clinical care.

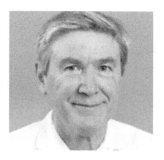

**PAUL DAVIES**
Email: paul.davies@asu.edu

Paul Davies is a theoretical physicist, cosmologist, astrobiologist and best-selling science author. He has published about 30 books and hundreds of research papers and review articles across a range of scientific fields. He is also well-known as a media personality and science popularizer in several countries. His research interests have focused mainly on quantum gravity, early universe cosmology, the theory of quantum black holes and the nature of time. He has also made important contributions to the field of astrobiology, and was an early advocate of the theory that life on Earth may have originated on Mars.

For several years he has also been running a major cancer research project, and developed a new theory of cancer based on tracing its deep evolutionary origins. Among his many awards are the 1995 Templeton Prize, the Faraday Prize from The Royal Society, the Kelvin Medal and Prize from the Institute of Physics, the Robinson Cosmology Prize and the Bicentenary Medal of Chile. He was made a member of the Order of Australia in the 2007 Queen's birthday honours list and the asteroid 6870 Pauldavies is named after him. His more recent books include "What's Eating the Universe," "The Demon in the Machine", "About Time", "The Origin of Life", "The Goldilocks Enigma: Why Is the Universe Just Right for Life?", "How to Build a Time Machine" and "The Eerie Silence: Are We Alone in the Universe?"

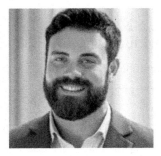

### JAKE BECRAFT

Jake Becraft is a Synthetic Biologist & Entrepreneur on a mission to advance the pace of innovation & accessibility of medicine.

He is Co-Founder & CEO @ Strand Therapeutics, and serves on its Board of Directors. Together with colleagues at MIT's renowned Synthetic Biology Center, he led the development of the world's first synthetic biology programming language for mRNA. Jake has been featured in Endpoints News, Fierce Biotech, Bloomberg, Forbes, and Business Insider, among others, for his vision and mission at Strand of applying this unique platform for real world disease applications.

He has also been the recipient of prestigious national and international awards for his scientific and entrepreneurial achievements, including the Barry Goldwater Scholarship and Excellence in Education Award, the Andrew Viterbi Fellowship of MIT, Amgen Fellowship, and the Bristol-Myers Squibb 2018 Golden Ticket for recognition of Strand as an innovative startup. Jake is a 2021 Termeer Fellow and has been named to MIT Tech Review's 35 Innovators under 35.

Jake is an outspoken advocate amongst the life science ecosystem for supporting young founders in entrepreneurship. Beyond Jake's work at Strand, his broader interests span synthetic biology, biologically engineered organism-machine interfaces, and the intersection of tech / bio methodologies. Currently, he serves on the Executive Board of Public Health

United, a non-profit focused on helping scientists better communicate their research for maximum impact. Previously, he served as a Science and Technology advisor to legislators in the Massachusetts State Legislature.

Outside of work, you can find Jake training in Brazilian Jiu Jitsu or heading to the mountains for some backcountry snowboarding.

Jake received his Ph.D. in Biological Engineering and Synthetic Biology from MIT and his B.S. in Chemical and Biomolecular Engineering from the University of Illinois at Urbana-Champaign, graduating Magna cum Laude with distinction.

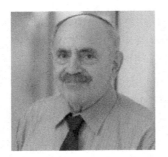

**ROBERT WEINBERG**
Email: weinberg@wi.mit.edu

Robert A. Weinberg studies how cancer spreads, what gives cancer stem-cells their unique qualities, and the molecular players involved in the formation of cancer stem cells and metastases.

We investigate three broad questions related to the origin and spread of cancer. First, how do cancer cells within a primary tumor acquire the ability to invade and metastasize? Second, how are the stem-cell state and the epithelial-mesenchymal transition interrelated? Third, how are the regulators of the epithelial-mesenchymal transition able to activate this profound change in cell phenotype?

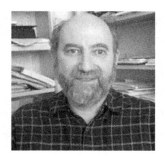

**STEVEN N. FIERING**
Email:
steven.n.fiering@dartmouth.edu

The immune system recognizes cancers and many are eliminated before they are clinically recognized. Cancer can be considered to be a failure of the immune system and it is now becoming clear that this immune failure is often due to active immunosuppression generated by the tumor. One approach to cancer therapy is finding ways to stimulate the immune system to seek out and destroy tumor cells much like it seeks out and destroys infectious organisms.

Our lab is currently focused on developing novel approaches to boosting anti-tumor immunity by injection of immune stimulatory reagents directly into recognized tumors, an approach termed "in situ vaccination". The goal is to overcome the local immunosuppression, get an effective local antitumor immune response and generate a systemic antitumor immune response to fight metastatic disease. All vaccines include an antigen to be recognized by the immune system and an adjuvant to stimulate the response against the antigen.

For in situ vaccination the tumor carries all relevant antigens and injection of adjuvant into the tumor supports recognition of both tumor-associated and neoantigens expressed by the tumor. There are many options to how in situ vaccination can be performed and we explore the options in mice as well as working with dogs with spontaneous tumors and studying the local and systemic immune response involved. The goal is to develop clinically useful in situ vaccination approaches.

Dr. Fiering received his Bachelor of Science from the University of Michigan in 1975, and his Doctorate from Stanford in 1990. After postdoctoral work as an NIH research fellow and research associate at the Fred Hutchinson Cancer Research Center, Dr. Fiering joined the faculty of the Department of Microbiology at Dartmouth Medical School in 1997.

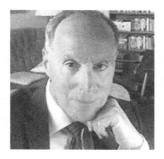

**RONALD B. BROWN**
Email: r26brown@uwaterloo.ca

Ronald B. Brown, PhD: He has authored over a dozen peer-reviewed articles in the U.S. National Library of Medicine of the National Institutes of Health; as well as a chapter on breakthrough knowledge synthesis in Contemporary Natural Philosophy and Philosophies.

In addition to his epidemiologic research on infectious disease and vaccines during the COVID-19 pandemic, his current areas of research include prevention of cancer, cardiovascular disease, dementia, and other chronic diseases. You can read his paper, "Phosphate Toxicity and Tumorigenesis" at ScienceDirect.com.

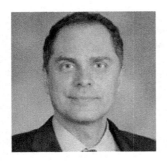

**DORU PAUL**

Email: dop9054@med.cornell.edu

My main goal as an oncologist is to improve the quality and the duration of life of my patients and, all through their treatment, to develop an environment of compassion and mutual trust. Research in oncology is crucial for improving the prognosis of cancer patients and I have a strong passion for clinical and translational research. Each person is different and I am constantly striving to provide my patients the best personalized oncology care currently available for his or her specific condition. Additionally, I am committed to integrating innovative and more performant diagnostic and treatment methods within my practice.

Dr. Paul is an expert in the treatment of head and neck and lung cancer with a track record of developing successful multidisciplinary approaches to treat these conditions. He has also made major contributions as a translational and clinical researcher. Demonstrating a national and international presence in his field, he has widely presented his research defining specific therapeutic targets or processes that can be targeted for the improved treatment of cancer patients.

Dr. Paul received his MD from the Carol Davila Faculty of Medicine in Bucharest, Romania and his PhD from the Faculty of Medicine in Craiova, Romania. He also got diplomas in Clinical Oncology, Chronobiology and Biology of Aging from Paris, France and he completed his training in Internal Medicine, Hematology and Medical Oncology in New York. Dr. Paul is an experienced clinician with more than ten thousand cancer patients treated until now and with a strong background in basic and translational research. He has designed and conducted several investigator-initiated studies and initiated three FDA approved investigational new drug studies including the first in-man pilot study that uses [18F] Fluorodeoxyglucose (FDG) for the targeted treatment of cancer. Since 2015, he has been working on a novel cancer model [see, for example "The systemic hallmarks of cancer" (2020) and "Cancer as a form of life: Musings of the cancer and evolution symposium" (2021). He is also the senior oncology editor of the verywellhealth.com website and the editor-in-chief of the Journal of Medical and Radiation Oncology.

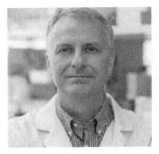

**MATTHEW VANDER HEIDEN**

Email: mvh@mit.edu,
pejansen@mit.edu

Mathew Vander Heiden is Professor in the Department of Biology and Director of the Koch Institute at MIT. He is also a member of the Broad Institute. He is a practicing oncologist and instructor in medicine at Dana-Farber Cancer Institute / Harvard Medical School. He earned his doctoral and medical degrees from the University of Chicago, where he worked in the laboratory of Craig Thompson. Vander Heiden then completed a residency in internal medicine at Boston's Brigham & Women's Hospital and a hematology-oncology fellowship at Dana-Farber Cancer Institute / Massachusetts General Hospital. He was a postdoctoral fellow in the laboratory of Lewis Cantley at Harvard Medical School, where he was supported by a Mel Karmazin Fellowship from the Damon Runyon Cancer Research Foundation.

In 2010, Vander Heiden joined the MIT faculty. His work has been recognized by many awards including the Burroughs Wellcome Fund Career Award for Medical Sciences, the AACR Gertrude B. Elion Award, an HHMI Faculty Scholar Award, and an NCI Outstanding Investigator Award. Dr. Vander Heiden serves on the scientific advisory board of Yale Cancer Center, the Salk Institute Cancer Center, the Wistar Institute Cancer Center, Agios Pharmaceuticals, iTeos Therapeutics, and Auron Therapeutics, of which he is also an academic founder. He is also part of the investment advisory board for DROIA Venture Fund.

## Research Summary

Cancer cells have metabolic requirements that differ from most normal, non-proliferating cells. To proliferate, cancer cells must transform available nutrients into the varied array of macromolecules that are needed to build a new cell. Each cancer type is unique and will have a metabolic phenotype that depends on tissue type, genetic factors, and local environment. How specific cancers integrate these factors and rewire their metabolism to support cancer progression is a major unanswered question.

The long-term goal of the Vander Heiden lab is to understand how mammalian cell metabolism is adapted to support cancer initiation and progression. The metabolic phenotypes of proliferating cells are typically interpreted with an emphasis on either energy generation or the crosstalk between signaling events and cell metabolism. This has led many to focus on how cancer genetics influence metabolic pathway use. The Vander Heiden lab takes a different approach that identifies limiting metabolic processes, considers how these are constrained by the extracellular environment, and defines how metabolic limitations are overcome within a physiological tissue context.

Using mass spectrometry to trace nutrient fate in cancer models, the Vander Heiden lab generates hypotheses for how different cancers use metabolism to support cell proliferation and tumor growth. They test these hypotheses using a variety of biochemical and genetic approaches to define how nutrient availability, metabolic pathway regulation, and tissue context constrain how cells use available materials to proliferate. The current interests of the laboratory include: 1) identifying which metabolic processes create bottlenecks for cell proliferation; 2) determining how metabolism is different in different cancers, examining in detail the influence of tissue type, tumor genetics, and tumor microenvironment; and 3) understanding how diet and whole body metabolism influence cell metabolism in tissues to modify cancer and other disease phenotypes. Through this work, they aim to advance understanding of metabolic pathway biochemistry and its relationship to cancer and mammalian physiology. Together, these studies will broaden our understanding of cancer cell metabolism will also identify approaches to target metabolism for cancer therapy.

Learn more about the Vander Heiden lab and their efforts to better understand cancer cell metabolism and how small molecules might be used to activate enzymes and restore the normal state of cells by watching this video: "Inside the Lab: Matthew Vander Heiden, M.D., Ph.D."

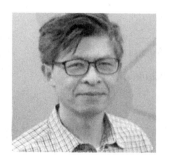

**SUI HUANG**

Email:
sui.huang@systemsbiology.org

Dr. Sui Huang is a molecular and cell biologist with a strong background in theoretical biology. He has devoted his research to understanding the very phenomenon of cancer from a complex systems perspective. Life scientists now readily acknowledge that the "whole is more than the sum of its parts" but the question is: What exactly is the "more" that we need in order to understand the "whole"? Can this abstract philosophical notion be reduced to a rigorous formal concept and concrete molecular entities?

Pursuing this question has guided Dr. Huang's research in cancer and cell biology over the past decade. Before joining the ISB in fall 2011, Dr. Huang held faculty positions at the University of Calgary (Institute of Biocomplexity and Informatics), where he helped establish biocomplexity as a discipline in research and teaching, and at Harvard Medical School (Children's Hospital) where he obtained first experimental evidence for the existence of high-dimensional attractors in mammalian gene regulatory networks.

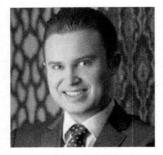

**ABDUL SLOCUM**
Email: abdulkadirsl@gmail.com

Dr. Abdul Kadir Slocum M.D. is originally from the United States but grew up in Istanbul, Turkey and completed his medical training at Marmara University, Istanbul. He comes from an integrative medical background and has a particular interest in helping patients suffering from cancer and exploring new ways of addressing the disease.

Fluent in both English and Turkish, since founding Chemothermia with Assistant Professor İyikesici and Professor Berkarda he has worked with them on the development and application of conventional as well as innovative treatment modalities for oncology and has particular responsibility for the clinic's international patients.

Chemothermia was founded in 2010 by two of the most experienced medical oncologists in Turkey: Prof. Bulent Berkada and Asst. Prof. Mehmet Salih İyikesici together with Dr Abdul Kadir Slocum, a leading proponent of integrative cancer care, in order to deliver world-class cancer treatment using the latest integrative approaches.

At Chemothermia, we are committed to expanding the paradigms for cancer treatment with the ultimate goal of creating a holistic treatment model which supports the patient whilst attacking the cancer, as opposed to attacking the cancer by attacking the patient. Our approach is grounded in the scientific study of the role of cellular metabolism in health – an overlooked area which is attracting increasing attention across the medical spectrum, from immunologists to mental health experts.

The fundamental premise of our approach is that cellular metabolism has a foundational role in all aspects of our health due to its role in regulating energy transference and balance throughout the body. Supporting and balancing this system against both the debilitations of cancer and of its treatment can increase the patient's resilience to both, giving them more time to fight the disease.

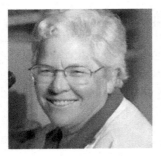

**ADRIENNE C. SCHECK**
Email: adrienne.scheck@gmail.com

Adrienne C. Scheck, PhD, is a Research Scientist in the Department of Child Health at the University of Arizona College of Medicine in Phoenix and in Neurodevelopmental Research at Phoenix Children's Hospital. She is also an Adjunct Professor at Arizona State University, an Associate Investigator in the Cancer Biology Program at the University of Arizona and an Adjunct Associate Professor the Barrow Neurological Institute (BNI). She received her BA from the University of Rochester and her PhD from Rensselaer Polytechnic Institute. After a postdoctoral fellowship in viral oncology at Pennsylvania State College of Medicine she moved to Sloan-Kettering Cancer Center to study AIDS-related dementia. Here she began studies of brain tumors and moved to the Barrow Neurological Institute in 1989 and remained there until 2017 when she moved to Phoenix Children's Hospital and the University of Arizona College of Medicine in Phoenix. Dr. Scheck is an acknowledged leader in the field of metabolic alteration as an adjunct to the standard of care to improve survival and minimize side effects for patients with malignant brain tumors. To this end, her laboratory has been studying the use of the therapeutic ketogenic diet (KD) and metabolic ketosis for the treatment of malignant brain tumors. Their work has shown that the KD reduces the growth of malignant brain tumors through a wide variety of mechanisms, and it potentiates the effect of radiation and temozolomide chemotherapy. She is now working to extend these studies to pediatric brain tumors. Dr. Scheck also has a strong interest in science education, and she has mentored over 150 students ranging from High School to Neurosurgical Fellows. In her free time, she enjoys spending time with her horses and cats.

**Research Interests**

Brain tumor diagnosis prognosis and therapy. Our main research focus is the modulation of metabolism for the adjuvant treatment of brain tumors.

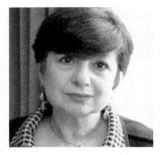

**ANA SOTO**
Email: ana.soto@tufts.edu

Dr. Ana M. Soto is a theoretical and experimental biologist. She is a professor at Tufts University School of Medicine, Boston, and a Fellow at the Centre Cavaillès, Ecole Normale Supérieure, Paris (ENS). She was the Blaise Pascal Chair in Biology 2013-15 at the ENS. Her research interests include the control of cell proliferation, the developmental origins of adult disease, the biomechanics of morphogenesis and theoretical and epistemological topics pertaining to biological organization. In this regard, in partnership with Professor Carlos Sonnenschein, she co-authored a book entitled THE SOCIETY OF CELLS (Bios-Springer-Verlag, 1999, published also in French in 2006, in Spanish in 2018 and it is now being translated to Italian).

They posited that the default state of cells in all organisms is proliferation, and proposed the Tissue Organization Field Theory of Carcinogenesis, in which cancer is viewed as development gone awry. As the Blaise Pascal Chair she coordinated a multidisciplinary working group devoted to the elaboration of a theory of organisms (Soto, AM, Longo, G Noble, D, editors: From the century of the genome to the century of the organism: New theoretical approaches. Prog. Biophys. Mol. Biol, 122:1, 2016).

Dr. Soto is the recipient of several awards, including the 2012 Gabbay Biotechnology & Medicine Award of Brandeis University, presented to her, Dr. Sonnenschein and Dr. Hunt as a result of their contributions to public health. She has been elected a member of the prestigious Collegium

Ramazzini, Carpi, Italy in 2011, and awarded the Blaise Pascal Chair of Biology 2013-15 at the Ecole Normale Supérieure, Paris. She was recently referenced in the article titled "The Top 50 Women in STEM" by TheBestSchools.org (https://thebestschools.org/features/50-top-women-in-stem/). In 2019 she was also awarded the Grand Vermeil Medal, the highest distinction from the City of Paris for her pioneering role in discovery endocrine disruptors.

Due to her unique profile spanning theoretical and experimental biology as well as public health issues she is frequently called to serve as member of government-sponsored advisory panels among them the US-National Academy of Sciences, Swiss National Science Foundation, US-EPA, EU-Environmental Agency. She has also been invited to testify before legislative bodies (US Congress, French Assemblée Nationale, etc).

Her research has been funded by the US National Science Foundation, the US-National Cancer Institute, the US EPA, the Susan G. Komen Foundation, the US-National Institute of Environmental Health Sciences, the Avon Foundation, the UK Medical Research Council, and EU research programs.

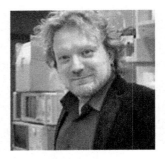

**ANDREAS MERSHIN**

Email: mershin@mit.edu

Andreas Mershin earned his MSci in Physics and Cosmology at Imperial College London and his PhD in Physics and Biophysics at Texas A&M University. He is currently a Research Scientist at the MIT Center for Bits and Atoms where he leads the Label Free Research Group that operates in blissful ignorance of any boundaries between physics, biology, materials and information sciences.

From inexpensive photosynthetic solar panels to quantum effects in molecular biology and from cytoskeletal memory encoding, machine olfaction to bioenergy harvesting, his research and the resulting technologies are used by industry and government, exhibited at the Boston Museum of Science and Designer's Open Exhibition and have been globally covered by CNN, BBC, NYT, Discovery Channel, Wired, New Scientist, Nature and Science.

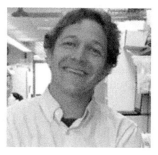

**BENJAMIN HOPKINS**

Email:
benjamin.hopkins@mssm.edu

Benjamin D. Hopkins, PhD, Assistant Professor of Genomics and Genetic Sciences, and Oncological Sciences, is the co-leader of the Functional Genomics Pipeline at The Tisch Cancer Institute. Dr. Hopkins and his team work to design and run precision medicine workflows, in order to facilitate translational cancer research at Mount Sinai. The Functional Genomics Pipeline focuses on two primary screening modalities. First, using an automated high-throughput screening platform developed by Dr. Hopkins for the Functional Genomics Pipeline, the group works to identify tumor specific drug sensitivities. Second, for new compounds or targets the group runs "inverse" screens to identify patient populations which are most likely to respond to a given therapy. Both of these screening modalities are run on three-dimensional organoid models developed in the laboratory from patients at Mount Sinai Hospital.

Dr. Hopkins studies cellular signaling with an emphasis on how systemic metabolism regulates key oncogenic pathways, such as the PI3K/PTEN signaling cascade. The overarching goal of the Hopkins Laboratory is to understand the molecular mechanisms that lead to drug sensitivities so that they can be leveraged in the clinic to improve patient outcomes. His group focuses on Breast, Lung, and Pancreatic cancer. The laboratory is comprised of a mix of computational and cell biologists.

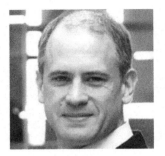

**CARLO MALEY**
Email: maley@asu.edu,
cbaciu@asu.edu

Carlo Maley is a cancer biologist, evolutionary biologist, and computational biologist, working at the intersection of those fields. He directs the Arizona Cancer Evolution Center at Arizona State University.

His team uses tools from evolution and ecology to help solve four problems in cancer: a) they use evolutionary and ecological measures of neoplasms to distinguish high from low-risk tumors, b) they develop new approaches for delaying or deflecting the evolutionary trajectories of premalignant neoplasms to prevent cancer, c) they develop methods to prevent or control the evolution of therapeutic resistance in cancers, d) they seek to discover the mechanisms that have evolved to suppress cancer in large, long-lived animals like elephants and whales, a problem known as Peto Paradox.

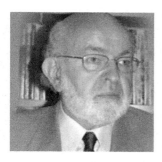

**CARLOS SONNENSCHEIN**

Email:
carlos.sonnenschein@tufts.edu

For over four decades, under the sponsorship of the NIH and other funding agencies, Dr. Ana M. Soto and I have worked on a) the control of the proliferation of estrogen- and androgen-target cells and b) carcinogenesis. These basic biological subjects are being explored under the fundamental premise that proliferation is the default state of all living cells and that cancer is a tissue-based disease, respectively. We have identified several plasma-borne and endogenously generated inhibitors of cell proliferation.

Over two decades ago, we proposed the tissue organization field theory of carcinogenesis (TOFT), which proposes that carcinogenesis is a tissue-based phenomenon. This notion challenges the one embodied in the hegemonic somatic mutation theory of carcinogenesis (SMT), which posits instead, that an accumulation of mutations in a single cell is responsible for the causation of a neoplasia.

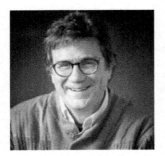

**CHARLEY LINEWEAVER**

Email:
charley.lineweaver@anu.edu.au

I have about a dozen projects dealing with exoplanet statistics, the recession of the Moon, cosmic entropy production, major transitions in cosmic and biological evolution and phylogenetic trees.

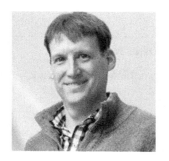

**DAVID GOODE**
Email: david.goode@petermac.org

The Goode laboratory combines bioinformatics, genomics, molecular evolution and population genetics to study the evolutionary forces governing the formation of tumours and their responses to therapy, with an emphasis on the roles of genomic instability and transcriptional plasticity as drivers of drug resistance in cancer. Our work centres mainly on prostate cancer and brain cancer, though our approaches are applicable to a range of solid tumours. Evolutionary genomics is the use of genome-scale analysis to investigate how natural selection has shaped genetic and phenotypic diversity between and within species.

As cancer results from strong selection for particular cellular phenotypes, evolutionary genomics has great potential to unlock the secrets of this disease. We use evolutionary genomics to study all stages of tumour evolution, through in-depth analysis of large genome and RNA sequencing data sets from cancer patients and laboratory models of cancer, along with computational and statistical modelling.

Our research involves assessing genetic, transcriptomic and phenotypic changes in individual tumours over time, as well as the impact impacts of mutation, selection and drift at the population and species level on the incidence and manifestation of cancer. We are particularly interested in the processes that generate genetic and transcriptional diversity within tumour and how these are shaped by external selective pressures.

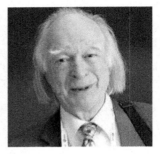

**DENIS NOBLE**
Email: denis.noble@dpag.ox.ac.uk

Denis Noble developed the first mathematical model of cardiac cells in 1960 using his discovery, with his supervisor Otto Hutter, of two of the main cardiac potassium ion channels. These discoveries were published in Nature (1960) and The Journal of Physiology (1962). The work was later developed with Dick Tsien, Dario DiFrancesco, Don Hilgemann and others to become the canonical models on which more than 100 cardiac cell models are based today. All are available on the CellML website.

He was elected President of the International Union of Physiological Sciences (IUPS) at its Congress in Kyoto in 2009, and the opening speech is available as a pdf on this page. He was then elected for a second term at the 2013 Congress in Birmingham, UK. He also delivered the opening plenary lecture at the Congress (see Music of Life link) which is also published as an article in Experimental Physiology (2013).

He is the author of the first popular book on Systems Biology, The Music of Life, and his most recent lectures concern the implications for evolutionary biology. To follow the debate on this see the FAQ (Answers) pages on the Music of Life website.

Denis Noble has published more than 500 papers and 11 books.

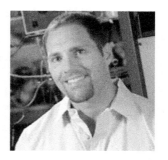

**DOMINIC D'AGOSTINO**
Email: ddagosti@usf.edu

The primary focus of our laboratory is developing and testing metabolic-based therapies, including ketogenic diets, ketone body supplements and metabolic-based drugs. Our laboratory uses in vivo and in vitro techniques to understand the physiological, cellular and molecular mechanism of metabolic therapies. Our research is supported by the Office of Naval Research (ONR), Department of Defense (DoD), private organizations, foundations and donations to USF.

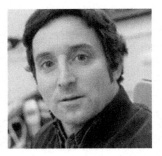

**FRANOIS FUKS**
Email: ffuks@ulb.ac.be

Fuks' lab hosts the Next-Generation Sequencing (NGS) platform dedicated to epigenomics (EPICS, EPIgenomic Creative Solutions). His group has an internationally recognized expertise in epigenomic analyses. Importantly, the key expertise in Infinium Methylation technology, was developed in collaboration with the major NGS Company, Illumina. Several national and international collaborations are ongoing through this technological platform. Thanks to EPICS, a biomarkers signature based on DNA methylation that measures the pre-existing immune response in a patient's tumor has been developed to discriminate breast cancer responders from non-responders to chemotherapy.

François has been acknowledged for his remarkable contribution to epigenetics with several awards, including the Lambertine Lacroix Foundation Award (2014) and Gaston Ithier Foundation Awards. He was the first recipient of the prestigious EMBO Young Investigator (YIP) Award (2007). He was also the recipient of the Young Investigator awards from the Wouters Foundation (2004) and from the Foundation Against Cancer (2001).

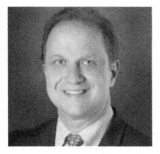

**GEORGE CALIN**
Email: gcalin@mdanderson.org

George Adrian Calin received both his M.D. and Ph.D. degrees at Carol Davila University of Medicine in Bucharest, Romania. After working in cytogenetics as an undergraduate student with Dragos Stefanescu in Bucharest, Calin completed cancer genomics training in Massimo Negrini's laboratory at the University of Ferrara, Italy, and in 2000, he became a postdoctoral fellow in Carlo Croce's laboratory at Kimmel Cancer Center in Philadelphia, Pennsylvania.

In June 2007, Calin joined MD Anderson as an associate professor in the Experimental Therapeutics department and was promoted to Professor with tenure in 2013. He explores new RNA therapeutic options for cancer patients and studies the roles of microRNAs and other non-coding RNAs in cancer initiation and progression, as well as the mechanisms of cancer predisposition.

Dr. Calin's main research interests are: 1) the involvement of non-coding RNAs in human diseases in general and of microRNAs in human cancers in particular, 2) the study of familial predisposition to human cancers, 3) the identification of ncRNA biomarkers in body fluids, and 4) the development of new RNA-based therapeutic options for cancer patients.

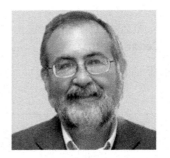

**HERBERT LEVINE**

Email: h.levine@northeastern.edu

Physical modeling of cancer progression, metastasis and interaction with the immune system. Most recent interests include the role of metabolic plasticity in these processes and the co-evolution of the tumor and the adaptive immune system.

Other areas include spatial organization of the actin cytoskeleton, the mechanics of collective cell motility, and the analysis of genetic circuits involved in cell fate decisions.

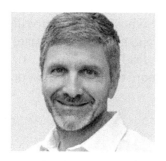

**JAMES DEGREGORI**
Email:
james.degregori@cuanschutz.edu

Our lab seeks to understand how carcinogenic conditions promote cancer evolution and to discover pathway dependencies in cancers that can be exploited therapeutically.

For the former, we have developed an evolutionary based model for cancer development, Adaptive Oncogenesis. In this model, mutations (including oncogenic mutations) face fitness landscapes that vary with age or following carcinogen exposure. We propose that long-lived multicellular organisms have evolved stem cell populations with high fitness, not only as a means of efficiently maintaining a tissue, but also because high fitness in a cell population will oppose somatic evolution. Highly effective competition in a young healthy stem cell population serves to maintain the status quo, preventing somatic evolution.

But in stem cell pools damaged by aging, irradiation or other insults, the fitness landscape will be dramatically altered. The fitness of the stem cell pool will be reduced, promoting selection for mutations and epigenetic events that improve fitness. Using mouse models and focusing on hematopoietic and lung tissues, we are currently exploring how reduced progenitor cell fitness resulting from aging and other insults can select for adaptive oncogenic events and thereby promote the expansion and fixation of oncogenically initiated cells.

Other studies in the lab are geared towards the development of novel therapeutic strategies to treat leukemias. We perform genome-wide loss-of-function screens using RNA interference

(RNAi) and CRISPR to identify genes whose inhibition will synergize with current targeted therapeutics to eliminate leukemia cells. These studies could lead to discovery of adjuvants to current therapies that will more effectively treat or possibly even cure leukemias.

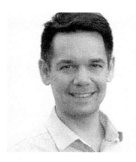

**Jo Bhakdi**
Email: jb@quantgene.com,
rachel@quantgene.com

Jo Bhakdi is the founder and CEO of Quantgene. His work in machine learning, sequencing technology, and DNA extraction procedures defines the cutting edge of genomic diagnostics, early disease detection, and precision medicine. Prior to Quantgene, Jo founded i2X, an investment framework that composes low-risk Venture Capital portfolios across large numbers of technology startups.

The i2X platform laid important foundations for advanced analytics in both financial and biotechnology applications, such as the Quantgene machine learning platform. Bhakdi holds a Masters in Economics and Psychology from Tubingen University, one of Germany's leading academic institutions, with a focus on financial theory and statistics.

He kicked off his career at WPP and Omnicom, where he held Strategy and Executive Director positions. Beyond his focus on technology and the future of medicine, Bhakdi is dedicated to bringing together the best and brightest and transforming them into pioneers, pushing the boundaries of health, life, and innovation for all.

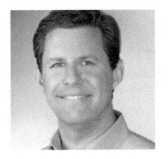

**JOSH OFMAN**
Email: kgrossman@grailbio.com,
jofman@grailbio.com

Josh Ofman, MD, MSHS, is Chief Medical Officer and External Affairs at GRAIL. Josh also serves on the Board of Directors of Cell BT, Inc, an immuno-therapy company focused on the discovery and development of innovative cancer therapeutics. Previously, Josh spent more than 15 years at Amgen, where he most recently held the role of Senior Vice President, Global Health Policy.

Prior to that, Josh was a faculty member in the Department of Medicine and Health Services Research at University of California, Los Angeles (UCLA) School of Medicine, Cedars-Sinai Medical Center, as well as Senior Vice President of Zynx Health Inc., a subsidiary of Cerner Corp. Josh holds a BA in history and philosophy of science from the University of California, Berkeley, and an MD from the University of California, Irvine, School of Medicine. Josh also has an MSHS from the UCLA School of Public Health.

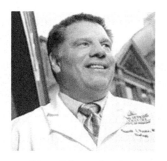

**KENNETH PIENTA**

Email: dlabuda@jhmi.edu,
kpienta1@jhmi.edu

Dr. Pienta's laboratory focuses on defining the tumor microenvironment of prostate cancer metastases and the development of new therapies for prostate cancer. These insights have been used to identify novel targets for the treatment of advanced prostate cancer, thus successfully moving bench research into the clinic in the form of Phase II and Phase III clinical trials. Currently, the lab operates under the hypothesis that there is an opportunity to devise new cancer therapies based on the recognition that tumors have properties of ecological systems.

There has been an increasing recognition that the tumor microenvironment contains host non-cancer cells in addition to cancer cells, interacting in a dynamic fashion over time. The cancer cells compete and/or cooperate with nontumor cells, and the cancer cells may compete and/or cooperate with each other. The interaction of these cancer and host cells to remodel the normal host organ microenvironment may best be conceptualized as an evolving ecosystem. We have used microdevices to help design ecosystems to mimic organ niches, such as bone marrow, that cancer cells metastasize to. Describing tumors as these ecological systems defines new opportunities for novel cancer therapies.

Dr. Kenneth J. Pienta is the Donald S. Coffey Professor of Urology and Professor of Oncology and Pharmacology and Molecular Sciences at the Johns Hopkins University School of Medicine and currently serves as the Director of Research for the The James Buchanan Brady Urological

Institute. He is a two-time American Cancer Society Clinical Research Professor Award recipient.

Dr. Pienta has an established peer-reviewed track record for organizing and administering a translational research program that successfully incorporates bench research, agent development, and clinical application. He has authored more than 350 peer-reviewed articles, has served as the Director of the Prostate Specialized Program of Research Excellence (SPORE) at The University of Michigan, and has led numerous local and national clinical trials. To date, Dr. Pienta has mentored more than 40 students, residents, and fellows to successful medical careers.

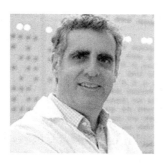

**MANEL ESTELLER**

Email:
emarin@carrerasresearch.org,
mesteller@carrerasresearch.org

From October 2001 to September 2008 Manel Esteller was the Leader of the CNIO Cancer Epigenetics Laboratory, where his principal areas of research were alterations in DNA methylation, histone modifications and chromatin in human cancer. He continued research in this field as the Director of the Cancer Epigenetics and Biology Program (PEBC) in the Bellvitge Biomedical Campus of Barcelona for ten years.

In May 2019, Dr Esteller became the Director of the Josep Carreras Leukaemia Research Institute (IJC) in Badalona (Barcelona). He is also Chairman of Genetics at the School of Medicine of the University of Barcelona, and an ICREA Research Professor. His current research is devoted to the establishment of the epigenome and epitranscriptome maps for normal and transformed cells, the study of the interactions between epigenetic modifications and non-coding RNAs, and the development of new epigenetic drugs for cancer therapy.

He is the author of more than 500 original publications in peer-reviewed scientific journals, 24 of them categorized as "Highly Cited Paper"s by Thomson Reuters, he is among the most cited researchers in the world (top 1%) with the recognition "Highly Cited Researcher" (decade 2008-2018) by Clarivate Analytics. He is also a Member of numerous international scientific societies and Editorial Boards and a reviewer for many journals and funding agencies. Dr Esteller is also the Associate Editor for Cancer Research, The Lancet Oncology, Carcinogenesis, Genome Research and The

Journal of The National Cancer Institute. He is the Editor-in-Chief of Epigenetics.

His work has received many awards including: , the Carcinogenesis Award (2005), the Beckman-Coulter Award (2006), the Fondazione Piemontese per la Ricerca sul Cancro (FPRC) Award (2006), the Swiss Bridge Award (2006), the Innovation Award from the Commonwealth of Massachussets (2007), the Human Frontier Science Program Award (2007), the DEbiopharm-EPFL Award (2009), the Dr. Josef Steiner Cancer Research Award (2009), the Lilly Foundation Preclinical Biomedical Research Award (2009), the World Health Summit Award (2010), the European Research Council Advanced Grant (2011), the "Rey Jaime I" Research Award (2013), the Severo Ochoa Award in Biomedicine (2014), the National Award in Oncology (2014), the "Dr Josep Trueta Medal" Goverment of Catalonia (2015), the National Research Award of the Government of Catalonia (2015), the Gold Medal of the Government of Catalonia (2016), the International Award of Catalonia (2016), the Falcó Carlemany Award (2017) and the Innovation in Healthcare Oncology Award (2018).

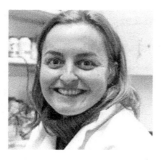

**MARIA CASANOVA-ACEBES**
Email: maria.casanova-acebes@mssm.edu

Maria is a postdoctoral fellow from Madrid, Spain. She received her PhD in Cellular Biology and Genetics under the supervision of Dr. Andrés Hidalgo at the Universidad Autónoma de Madrid (Spain) in 2015. Her PhD studies were focused on understanding the mechanisms of neutrophil aging and how the natural clearance of aged neutrophils triggers the homeostatic release of hematopoietic progenitors from bone marrow into the blood.

She joined Dr. Merad laboratory in April 2015, after being awarded a long-term postdoctoral fellowship from the Human Frontiers Science Program. During her postdoctoral research she is currently interested in the role of macrophage ontogeny in the context of lung adenocarcinoma progression in primary tumors.

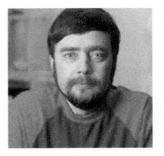

**MICHAEL LEVIN**
Email: michael.levin@tufts.edu

I was always interested in artificial intelligence and philosophy of mind - trying to understand how the biological world harnesses the laws of physics to create its remarkable living creatures. I received dual BS degrees in computer science and Biology from Tufts (1988-1992), and then a PhD in genetics from Harvard (1992-1996). Following a post-doc at Harvard Medical School, I started my independent lab in 200 at the Forsyth Institute (Harvard School of Dental Medicine) and then moved the group over to Tufts in 2009.

I am currently Distinguished Professor of Biology, holding the Vannevar Bush chair and serving as the director of the Allen Discovery Center at Tufts. My group works on living tissues as computational systems - as multi-scale agents which process information during embryogenesis, regeneration, and cancer. We use tools and concepts from biophysics, machine learning, and cognitive science to understand how cells communicate and form collectives that pursue large-scale goals - creation and repair of complex anatomies.

Our unique focus is on bioelectrical signals, by means of which all cells (not just neurons) form networks that process morphological information, regulate gene expression, and make decisions about dynamic growth and form. We have learned to listen in on these bioelectric conversations, and manipulate the electrically-encoded pattern memories (using molecular methods) for applications like repairing birth defects, inducing limb regeneration, and normalizing tumors. We use the insights of computer science to help us understand how cells and tissues process information, and conversely, use our biological discoveries to shed light on how new cognitive architectures can be created that are based on ancient primitive problem-solving capacities of all cells, not just o brains. Our most recent work concerns the creation of synthetic living machines - novel bodies made of various kinds of cells that self-organize new body shapes and behaviors.

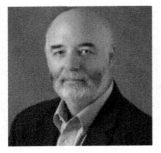

**PATRICK S. MOORE**
Email: psm9@pitt.edu

Our lab investigates viral causes of human malignancy and identifies new cancer-causing viruses using digital transcriptome subtraction. We currently focus on two agents we have discovered, KSHV (the viral cause of Kaposi's sarcoma) and MCV (the viral cause for most Merkel cell carcinomas). We focus on the basic molecular virology of transformation as well as develop assays that have clinical value in detecting tumor virus infection.

Most recently, we have characterized MCV mutations that truncate the MCV T antigen helicase to disable viral replication in tumors. We have also developed MCV T antigen monoclonal antibodies and virus-like particle serologic tests that allow us to screen patients and tissues for MCV infection. Additional research involves the search for potential KSHV vaccine candidates through analysis of latent KSHV protein immune processing.

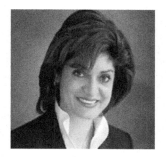

**RABIA BHATTI**
Email: rabia.bhatti@me.com

Medical school- Aga Khan University Medical College Karachi Pakistan 1988 Research fellow at St. Mary's Hospital London, UK 1990 and Loyola University 1991.

Metropolitan Group hospitals residency in general surgery 1998. Board certified general surgeon Assistant clinical professor of surgery Midwestern University Fellowship in Integrative Medicine from University of Arizona with Dr. Andrew Weil. Devote my time to taking care of breast cancer patients using national standards. Set up the multidisciplinary breast centers at West Suburban Medical Center, Oak Park and at Amita Resurrection Medical Center where a team of physicians, navigator, social worker works together to take holistic care of breast cancer patients.

Am passionate about breast cancer prevention and wellness and spend time doing community lectures. I practice what I preach and am an avid hiker and workout regularly. Also I am interested in teaching younger generation of surgeons in training to become skillful, knowledgeable and compassionate physicians and surgeons. I am my patient's strongest advocate. My philosophy is to treat my patients just as I would want my family members to be treated. I want to inform and educate my patients, so they become partners with me in their journey from breast cancer diagnosis to treatment.

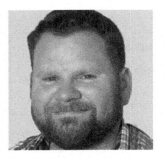

**RICHARD WHITE III**
Email: raw937@gmail.com

The bedrock of his work is how "viral lifestyles,' (i.e., whether lytic or lysogenic) in bacteriophage (viruses that infect bacteria) impacts the 'guts' of humans, plants (e.g., the rhizosphere), and modern microbialites. He has recently returned to his roots of molecular virology of human viruses by tackling COVID-19 and other RNA viruses (e.g., Influenza and Henipavirus) by targeting replication mechanisms with novel protein-based therapies. The goal of the work is to produce universal antivirals for RNA viruses in humans and animals. As well as my lab (the RAW lab) will tackle multidrug-resistant bacteria using bacteriophage therapy.

'The goal of our work is to make COVID-19 the last pandemic and stop the next major health crisis of multidrug-resistant bacteria.'

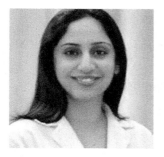

**RUCHI GABA**
Email: ruchi.gaba@bcm.edu

Dr. Ruchi Gaba obtained her medical degree from University College of Medical Sciences (UCMS) in New Delhi, India followed by residency in Internal Medicine at University of Alabama at Birmingham (UAB) and then fellowship in Endocrinology, Diabetes and Metabolism at Baylor College of Medicine (BCM) and has been faculty at BCM since 2015.

Her clinical expertise include evaluation and treatment of patients with endocrine neoplasia especially advanced thyroid cancer in addition to a variety of complicated thyroid disorders like hyperthyroidism, hypothyroidism, thyroid nodules/FNA and thyroid ds in pregnancy. She takes care of these patients with a multidisciplinary team including surgery, ENT, radiology, nuclear medicine and pathology. She also has vast clinical experience in taking care of patients with Atypical Diabetes like Ketosis Prone Diabetes and nonalcoholic fatty liver disease (NAFLD) and is actively involved in cutting edge research in the same. She is well recognized by her patients for utmost compassion, calm demeanor and great bedside manners.

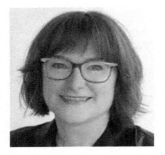

**SAMANTHA BUCKTROUT**

Email: sbucktrout@parkerici.org,
jinfanti@parkerici.org

Samantha Bucktrout Ph.D. is the Senior Director of Research at PICI. She is a cellular immunologist who applies discovery, translational and clinical datasets to transformative research and clinical studies. Samantha supports the strategy of PICI to have significant impact on the use and understanding of cancer immunotherapies. She has an extensive track record of collaborative research and leadership. Samantha built and leads the PICI brain tumor initiative, in collaboration with institute members interprets and elevates basic and clinical research in immune-therapy-resistant tumor types and immunotherapy discovery and development.

She co-leads development of a novel oncolytic virus for solid tumor therapy and has established collaborations with leading tumor-immune profiling technology groups for basic research and translational medicine. Samantha applies her expertise in cancer immunology and autoimmunity, leading research efforts in the mechanistic understandings of immune-related adverse events and has established and leads a research consortium for germline genetics in cancer immunotherapy. She is an active member of the PICI diversity, equity, inclusion and belonging committee, and leads the BIPOC internship program.

Prior to joining PICI, Samantha headed an immunotherapy research and development group at Pfizer Inc. for cancer and autoimmune indications. The focus of her research was patient T cell biology andmodulation by protein therapeutics. Samantha's pre-clinical research expertise was garnered with two postdoc positions in groups of leading immunologists: The Bluestone Laboratory at UCSF and The Miller Laboratory at Northwestern University. Her research uncovered novel facets of T cell and dendritic cell biology that establish setpoints of immune tolerance and autoimmunity. She has co-authored numerous book chapters, scientific reviews, patent applications and peer reviewed manuscripts. Samantha earned her Bachelor of Biology from the University of Aberdeen, Scotland, and Ph.D. in Immunology from the University of Edinburgh, Scotland, U.K.

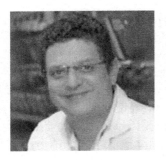

**SAMUEL SIDI**

Email: samuel.sidi@mssm.edu

Cancer target discovery in zebrafish (genetic and chemical-genetic approaches), mechanism of action of targeted therapies, development of molecular diagnostics. For more information, please visit the Sidi Laboratory. The Sidi Laboratory is focusing on Cancer Target Discovery in Zebrafish.

We exploit the whole-animal and high-throughput capacity of the zebrafish embryo, together with validation studies in human cancer cells to uncover cellular proteins/pathways that become essential in the presence of specific cancer mutations. The goal is to define novel, safer targets for systemic inhibitions in patients.

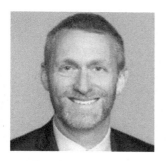

**SANDY BOROWSKY**

Email: adborowsky@ucdavis.edu, wiju@ucdavis.edu

Sandy Borowsky, MD, of the UC Davis Center for Comparative Medicine and the UC Davis Comprehensive Cancer Institute is an international leader in education and training in comparative pathology. As director of the Center for Genomic Pathology, centered at the University of California Davis, Dr. Borowsky is available to guide UCSF investigators and trainees to important educational and training opportunities.

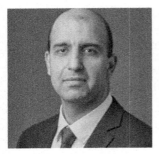

**SEYEDTAGHI TAKYAR**
Email: seyedtaghi.takyar@yale.edu

Shervin has a PhD in microbiology and molecular biology in The University of Queensland, Australia. During my PhD I worked and published on a variety of projects including developing a new lentiviral vector based on JDV (Jembrana Disease Virus), translational regulation in HCV by small RNA-binding molecules and the viral core protein, and RNA-protein interactions in positive strand RNA viruses. During this time I was also involved in cloning the Australian isolate of HCV with Dr Eric Gowans. My findings in these projects were published in a variety of journal including PNAS, Hepatology, and Journal of Molecular Biology. My next stop was a postdoctoral fellowship with Prof. Harry Noller at the RNA Center in UCSC where I delved deeper into the RNA world and studied the helicase activity of the ribosome during translation. Our work was well received and published in Cell.

I started my Internal Medicine residency at the State University of New York (SUNY) at Buffalo in 2003. During the last year of my residency I took part in a research project led by Dr Sands on the role of TIMP-1 in reactive airway disease. Our work was published in Clinical Immunology. I was then recruited to the Pulmonary Critical Care Fellowship at Yale in 2007, and worked with Dr J Elias to set up a platform for analyzing the role of microRNAs in the lung disease using the transgenic models that have been developed in his lab. I started this work on an inducible, lung-specific, VEGF transgenic model and within the first year of the project found a microRNA that was regulated by VEGF and mediated the effects of this cytokine in the lung. Based on these findings we filed a patent on the diagnostic and therapeutic use of miR-1 in lung disease. I received a K99/R00 award in the third year of my clinical fellowship for my work on this project. I was directly recruited as a tenure-track Assistant Professor in the Yale Pulmonary, Critical Care and Sleep Medicine Section at the end of my fellowship.

Since starting my tenure track position in 2010 I have been awarded the AAP (American Association of Physicians) Junior Investigator Award for my work on microRNAs in the lung and have given invited presentations at various international conferences. Our work on the role of VEGF-miR-1 axis in lung Th2 inflammation was published in Journal of Experimental Medicine. I successfully transitioned to the R00 (Independent investigator) phase of my NIH grant in 2013. I have recruited and worked with two postdoctoral fellows and three Associate Research Scientists over the last three years. My research currently focuses on the role of vascular non-coding RNAs in Th2 inflammation, lung injury and cancer.

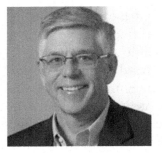

**STEVE GULLANS**
Email: steve.gullans@gmail.com

Steve is an experienced biotech executive, venture investor, scientist, entrepreneur, and author. He currently advises life science companies on strategy. Previously he was CEO of Gemphire Therapeutics, Inc., a public biotech which he joined after 10 years as a Managing Director at Excel Venture Management (EVM), a firm he co-founded and which invested $225M across more than 40 life science companies. At Excel, Steve served as a Board Director of more than a dozen private and public biotech, medtech, diagnostics, and health IT companies with many successful exits. Prior to Excel, Steve held CEO and CSO positions at two life sciences companies. Steve is currently a Director at Orionis Biosciences, Alexis Bio, Atentiv Health, iSpecimen, and Navigation Sciences.

Steve began his career as a professor at Harvard Medical School and Brigham & Women's Hospital where he published more than 130 scientific papers and was elected a Fellow of the American Association for the Advancement of Science and of the American Heart Association. He was an advisor to the Innovation Groups at the Cleveland Clinic and the Mass General Brigham. He received his Ph.D. from Duke University, post-doctoral training at Yale University, and his B.S. from Union College.

Steve loves innovation and has spoken widely, including at TED, TEDMED, and TEDx. With Juan Enriquez he co-authored Evolving Ourselves, a book that provides a sweeping tour of how humans are changing the course of evolution. Throughout his career he has focused on translating scientific advances into solutions for patients.

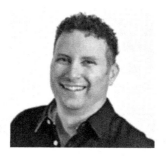

**STEVEN EISENBERG**
Email: steveneyes@gmail.com

In Dr. Steven Eisenberg's oncology practice, the enemy is cancer, but it's also denial, anger, and fear--draining emotions that can interfere with the effectiveness of treatment. Every day, Dr. Steven helps patients fight cancer using both time-tested conventional therapies and innovative medical technologies. At the same time, he helps them overcome negative emotions by cultivating acceptance, love, and self-compassion in a deeply personal way, through laughter, empathy, and the music he plays and sings for and with them.

How often do you hear someone say, "I'm alive"? Dr. Steven's patients say it to him all the time, in conversations, texts, and e-mails. Some of these patients are celebrating remissions or cures. Some are getting sicker, with reservations about what tomorrow might bring. But they've had a good day. They are all--we are all--truly and urgently alive. Dr. Steven's book invites us to celebrate this truth, even as it tells a compelling story of a doctor's experience on the front lines of care; offers a road map for bringing humanity back into traditional medical practice; and gives patients, families, and caregivers a blueprint for living each day with hope.

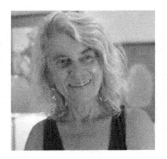

**SUSAN WADIA-ELLS**
Email:
susan@bustingbreastcancer.com

Susan Wadia-Ells is a long-time cultural change agent. During the 1970's she organized women at Polaroid, creating the first affirmative action program for women within a Fortune 200 corporation, and soon became Polaroid's corporate affirmative action manager and a mentor to other women's groups fighting for equal pay, training, benefits, and career opportunities.

After returning to academia in the early 1980's for a graduate degree in energy economics and political development at The Fletcher School, Dr. Wadia-Ells worked with community development groups in Zimbabwe as that nation's long struggle against apartheid ended. Next, she worked as a small town journalist in Brattleboro VT, under the guidance of the legendary UPI International Editor, Norman Runnion. Wadia-Ells then moved on to complete her PhD in women's studies, before teaching over the next decade in Lesley University's Adult Baccalaureate Program in Boston—helping women learn to fearlessly write their unspoken ideas and life stories.

During this time, while raising her son, she also created national feminist conferences on once-ignored or banned topics including the landmark Women's Ways of Knowing Study; exploring the psychological and spiritual dimensions within motherhood, and understanding the power of women's menopausal years.

Her 1995 anthology, *The Adoption Reader: Birth Mothers, Adoptive Mothers and Adopted Daughters Tell Their Stories*

(Seal Press, Seattle), helped define adoption as primarily a woman's issue. Wadia-Ells' column, "Honest Health", published by the Gloucester Daily Times (MA), beginning in 2008, her long-time Busting Breast Cancer blog, and her 2013 e-book, *Birth Control Drugs and Breast Cancer: Learn the Terrible Truth*, all served to introduce many of the topics discussed in her 2021 book, *Busting Breast Cancer: Five Simple Steps to Keep Breast Cancer out of Your Body*, based on the new metabolic theory of cancer. She currently lives in Manchester by the Sea, MA.

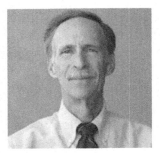

**WILLIAM MILLER**

Email: wbmiller1@cox.net

William B. Miller, Jr is the author of the book, "The Microcosm Within: Evolution and Extinction in the Hologenome". This work offers a complete alternative theory of evolution. Instead of the Darwinian belief in random genetic mutations and natural selection, Dr. Miller insists that evolution can only be properly understood through an approach that emphasizes an essential self-referential capacity that has defined all living things from its origin forward. All living entities use of information for communication, for collaboration, and to compete. All such actions are directed towards problem-solving to attain or sustain preferential conditions.

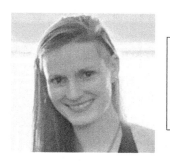

**LINDSAY HOESCHEN**
Editor, Speakeasy Marketing, Inc.
lindsay@speakeasymarketinginc.com

Five years of undergraduate study in philosophy and the sciences, and four years as a freelance writer and editor has taught Lindsay Hoeschen at least one solid lesson: when the cat walks across the keyboard more than once, it's obligatory break time.

Since graduating from Portland State University School of Honors in 2014, Lindsay has pursued myriad interests along a nonlinear path, but always with a steadfast loyalty to the practice of critical thinking, self-reflection, and creativity.

# REFERENCES

1. Shapiro JA. All living cells are cognitive. Biochemical and Biophysical Research Communications. 2021;564:134-149. doi:10.1016/j.bbrc.2020.08.120

2. Baluška F, Miller WB Jr. Senomic view of the cell: senome versus genome. Commun Integr Biol. 2018 Aug 10;11(3):1-9. doi: 10.1080/19420889.2018.1489184. PMID: 30214674; PMCID: PMC6132427.

3. Balakrishnan L, Milavetz B. Epigenetic regulation of viral biological processes. Viruses. 2017 Nov 17;9(11):346. doi: 10.3390/v9110346. PMID: 29149060; PMCID: PMC5707553.

4. Postat J, Bousso P. Quorum sensing by monocyte-derived populations. Front Immunol. 2019;10:2140. Published 2019 Sep 11. doi:10.3389/fimmu.2019.02140

5. Duddy OP, Bassler BL. Quorum sensing across bacterial and viral domains. PLoS Pathog. 2021;17(1):e1009074. Published 2021 Jan 7. doi:10.1371/journal.ppat.1009074

6. Gallagher J. More than half your body is not human. BBC News. https://www.bbc.com/news/health-43674270. Published April 10, 2018.

7. Grandi N, Tramontano E. Human endogenous retroviruses are ancient acquired elements still shaping innate immune responses. Front Immunol. 2018 Sep 10;9:2039. doi: 10.3389/fimmu.2018.02039. PMID: 30250470; PMCID: PMC6139349.

8. Mi S, Lee X, Li X, et al. Syncytin is a captive retroviral envelope protein involved in human placental morphogenesis. Nature. 2000;403(6771):785-789. doi:10.1038/35001608

9. Barford, E. Parasite makes mice lose fear of cats permanently. Nature (2013). https://doi.org/10.1038/nature.2013.13777

10. Enard D, Cai L, Gwennap C, Petrov DA. Viruses are a dominant driver of protein adaptation in mammals. eLife. 2016;5. doi:10.7554/elife.12469

11. Hunter P. We are what we eat. The link between diet, evolution and non-genetic inheritance. EMBO Rep. 2008;9(5):413-415. doi:10.1038/embor.2008.61

12. McAllister F, Khan MAW, Helmink B, Wargo JA. The tumor microbiome in pancreatic cancer: bacteria and beyond. Cancer Cell. 2019 Dec 9;36(6):577-579. doi: 10.1016/j.ccell.2019.11.004. PMID: 31951558.

13. Nowogrodzki, A. Tasmanian devils show signs of resistance to devastating facial cancer. Nature (2016). https://doi.org/10.1038/nature.2016.20508

14. Strakova, A., Murchison, E.P. The changing global distribution and prevalence of canine transmissible venereal tumour. BMC Vet Res 10, 168 (2014). https://doi.org/10.1186/s12917-014-0168-9

15. Heng J, Heng HH. Two-phased evolution: Genome chaos-mediated information creation and maintenance. Prog Biophys Mol Biol. 2021 Oct;165:29-42. doi: 10.1016/j.pbiomolbio.2021.04.003. Epub 2021 May 13. PMID: 33992670

16. Costanzo V, Bardelli A, Siena S, Abrignani S. Exploring the links between cancer and placenta development. Open Biol. 2018;8(6):180081. doi:10.1098/rsob.180081

17. Eigner, K., Filik, Y., Mark, F. et al. The unfolded protein response impacts melanoma progression by enhancing FGF expression and can be antagonized by a chemical chaperone. Sci Rep 7, 17498 (2017). https://doi.org/10.1038/s41598-017-17888-9

18. Yu L, Chen X, Wang L, Chen S. Oncogenic virus-induced aerobic glycolysis and tumorigenesis. J Cancer. 2018;9(20):3699-3706. Published 2018 Sep 8. doi:10.7150/jca.27279

19. Cooper GM. The Cell: A molecular approach. 2nd edition. Sunderland (MA): Sinauer Associates; 2000. The development and causes of cancer. Available from: https://www.ncbi.nlm.nih.gov/books/NBK9963/

20. Basu AK. DNA Damage, mutagenesis and cancer. Int J Mol Sci. 2018 Mar 23;19(4):970. doi: 10.3390/ijms19040970. PMID: 29570697; PMCID: PMC5979367.

21. Evans S, Campbell C, Naidenko OV. Cumulative risk analysis of carcinogenic contaminants in United States drinking water. Heliyon. 2019;5(9):e02314. doi:10.1016/j.heliyon.2019.e02314

22. Known and probable human carcinogens. Cancer.org. Published 2015. https://www.cancer.org/cancer/cancer-causes/general-info/known-and-probable-human-carcinogens.html

23. Sung H, Ferlay J, Siegel RL, et al. Global cancer statistics 2020: GLOBOCAN estimates of incidence and mortality worldwide for 36 cancers in 185 countries. CA: A Cancer Journal for Clinicians. 2021;71(3):209-249. doi:10.3322/caac.21660

24. DeGregori J. Connecting cancer to its causes requires incorporation of effects on tissue microenvironments. Cancer Res. 2017;77(22):6065-6068. doi:10.1158/0008-5472.CAN-17-1207

25. Seyfried TN. Cancer as a mitochondrial metabolic disease. Front Cell Dev Biol. 2015;3:43. Published 2015 Jul 7. doi:10.3389/fcell.2015.00043

26. Bulun SE, Chen D, Moy I, Brooks DC, Zhao H. Aromatase, breast cancer and obesity: a complex interaction. Trends Endocrinol Metab. 2012;23(2):83-89. doi:10.1016/j.tem.2011.10.003

27. What is phosphate and how is it used? | OCP Group. www.ocpgroup.ma. https://www.ocpgroup.ma/what-is-phosphate

28. Carpenter SR. Phosphorus control is critical to mitigating eutrophication. Proceedings of the National Academy of Sciences. 2008;105(32):11039-11040. doi:10.1073/pnas.0806112105

29. Brown RB, Razzaque MS. Phosphate toxicity and tumorigenesis. Biochim Biophys Acta Rev Cancer. 2018 Apr;1869(2):303-309. doi: 10.1016/j.bbcan.2018.04.007. Epub 2018 Apr 21. PMID: 29684520.

30. Chen S, Parmigiani G. Meta-analysis of BRCA1 and BRCA2 penetrance. J Clin Oncol. 2007 Apr 10;25(11):1329-33. doi: 10.1200/JCO.2006.09.1066. PMID: 17416853; PMCID: PMC2267287.

31. Szentgyorgyi A. The living state and cancer. Biophysics. 1977;74(7):2844-2847. Accessed December 4, 2021. https://www.pnas.org/content/pnas/74/7/2844.full.pdf

32. Yamashita M, Suda T. Low-dose X-rays leave scars on human hematopoietic stem and progenitor cells: the role of reactive oxygen species. Haematologica. 2020;105(8):1986-1988. doi:10.3324/haematol.2020.254292

33. Guinn MT, Wan Y, Levovitz S, Yang D, Rosner MR, Balázsi G. Observation and control of gene expression noise: barrier crossing analogies between drug resistance and metastasis. Frontiers in Genetics. 2020;11. doi:10.3389/fgene.2020.586726

34. Kumar P, Murphy FA. Who is this man? Francis Peyton Rous. Emerg Infect Dis. 2013;19(4):661-663. doi:10.3201/eid1904.130049

35. Javier RT, Butel JS. The history of tumor virology. Cancer Res. 2008;68(19):7693-7706. doi:10.1158/0008-5472.CAN-08-3301

36. Friend C. Cell-free transmission in adult Swiss mice of a disease having the character of a leukemia. J Exp Med. 1957;105(4):307-318. doi:10.1084/jem.105.4.307

37. Gross L. A filterable agent, recovered from Ak leukemic extracts, causing salivary gland carcinomas in C3H mice. Proc Soc Exp Biol Med. 1953 Jun;83(2):414-21. doi: 10.3181/00379727-83-20376. PMID: 13064287.

38. Pagano JS. Epstein-Barr virus: the first human tumor virus and its role in cancer. Proc Assoc Am Physicians. 1999 Nov-Dec;111(6):573-80. doi: 10.1046/j.1525-1381.1999.t01-1-99220.x. PMID: 10591086.

39. Kuri, A., Jacobs, B.M., Vickaryous, N. et al. Epidemiology of Epstein-Barr virus infection and infectious mononucleosis in the United Kingdom. BMC Public Health 20, 912 (2020). https://doi.org/10.1186/s12889-020-09049-x

40. Muñoz N, Castellsagué X, de González AB, Gissmann L. Chapter 1: HPV in the etiology of human cancer. Vaccine. 2006;24:S1-S10. doi:10.1016/j.vaccine.2006.05.115

41. Tashiro, H., Brenner, M. Immunotherapy against cancer-related viruses. Cell Res 27, 59–73 (2017). https://doi.org/10.1038/cr.2016.153

42. Ahuja, D., Sáenz-Robles, M. & Pipas, J. SV40 large T antigen targets multiple cellular pathways to elicit cellular transformation. Oncogene 24, 7729–7745 (2005). https://doi.org/10.1038/sj.onc.1209046

43. Schütze DM, Krijgsman O, Snijders PJ, et al. Immortalization capacity of HPV types is inversely related to chromosomal instability. Oncotarget. 2016;7(25):37608-37621. doi:10.18632/oncotarget.8058

44. Bryan TM, Reddel RR. SV40-induced immortalization of human cells. Crit Rev Oncog. 1994;5(4):331-57. doi: 10.1615/critrevoncog.v5.i4.10. PMID: 7711112.

45. Parkin DM. The global health burden of infection-associated cancers in the year 2002. International Journal of Cancer. 2006;118(12):3030-3044. doi:10.1002/ijc.21731

46. Vescovo T, Refolo G, Vitagliano G, Fimia GM, Piacentini M. Molecular mechanisms of hepatitis C virus–induced hepatocellular carcinoma. Clinical Microbiology and Infection. 2016;22(10):853-861. doi:10.1016/j.cmi.2016.07.019

47. Marx JL. Strong new candidate for AIDS agent. Science. 1984 May 4;224(4648):475-7. doi: 10.1126/science.6324344. PMID: 6324344.

48. Gonçalves PH, Uldrick TS, Yarchoan R. HIV-associated Kaposi sarcoma and related diseases. AIDS. 2017;31(14):1903-1916. doi:10.1097/QAD.0000000000001567

49. Gaston K. Small DNA Tumour Viruses. Accessed December 4, 2021. https://www.caister.com/hsp/prelims/dna-tumour-viruses.pdf

50. Poulin DL, DeCaprio JA. Is there a role for SV40 in human cancer? J Clin Oncol. 2006 Sep 10;24(26):4356-65. doi: 10.1200/JCO.2005.03.7101. PMID: 16963733.

51. Moore MJ, Sebastian JA, Kolios MC. Determination of cell nucleus-to-cytoplasmic ratio using imaging flow cytometry and a combined ultrasound and photoacoustic technique: a

comparison study. J Biomed Opt. 2019;24(10):1-10. doi:10.1117/1.JBO.24.10.106502

52. What do doctors look for in biopsy and cytology specimens? www.cancer.org. https://www.cancer.org/treatment/understanding-your-diagnosis/tests/testing-biopsy-and-cytology-specimens-for-cancer/what-doctors-look-for.html#:~:text=Size%20and%20shape%20of%20the%20cell

53. Nagy JA, Chang SH, Dvorak AM, Dvorak HF. Why are tumour blood vessels abnormal and why is it important to know?. Br J Cancer. 2009;100(6):865-869. doi:10.1038/sj.bjc.6604929

54. Zhang L, Yu D. Exosomes in cancer development, metastasis, and immunity. Biochim Biophys Acta Rev Cancer. 2019;1871(2):455-468. doi:10.1016/j.bbcan.2019.04.004

55. Anderson NM, Simon MC. The tumor microenvironment. Current Biology. 2020;30(16):R921-R925. doi:10.1016/j.cub.2020.06.081

56. Guernet A, Mungamuri S, Cartier D, et al. CRISPR-Barcoding for intratumor genetic heterogeneity modeling and functional analysis of oncogenic driver mutations. Molecular Cell. 2016;63(3):526-538. doi:10.1016/j.molcel.2016.06.017

57. Chen X, Wanggou S, Bodalia A, Zhu M, Dong W, Fan JJ, Yin W, Min H, Hu M, Draghici D, Dou W, Li F, Coutinho FJ, Whetstone H, Kushida MM, Dirks PB, Song Y, Hui C, Sun Y, Wang L, Li X, Huang X. A feedforward mechanism mediated by mechanosensitive ion channel PIEZO1 and Tissue Mechanics Promotes Glioma Aggression. Neuron. 2018;100(4):799-815.e7. doi:10.1016/j.neuron.2018.09.046 https://doi.org/10.1016/j.neuron.2018.09.046

58. Kornelia Polyak, MD, PhD - DF/HCC. www.dfhcc.harvard.edu. Accessed December 4, 2021. https://www.dfhcc.harvard.edu/insider/member-detail/member/kornelia-polyak-md-phd/

59. Manavathi B, Dey O, Gajulapalli VN, Bhatia RS, Bugide S, Kumar R. Derailed estrogen signaling and breast cancer: an authentic couple. Endocr Rev. 2013;34(1):1-32. doi:10.1210/er.2011-1057

60. Fernald K, Kurokawa M. Evading apoptosis in cancer. Trends Cell Biol. 2013;23(12):620-633. doi:10.1016/j.tcb.2013.07.006

61. Francescone R, Hou V, Grivennikov SI. Microbiome, inflammation, and cancer. Cancer J. 2014;20(3):181-189. doi:10.1097/PPO.0000000000000048

62. Li, Y., Tinoco, R., Elmén, L. et al. Gut microbiota dependent anti-tumor immunity restricts melanoma growth in Rnf5−/−mice. Nat Commun 10, 1492 (2019). https://doi.org/10.1038/s41467-019-09525-y

63. Maley, C., Aktipis, A., Graham, T. et al. Classifying the evolutionary and ecological features of neoplasms. Nat Rev Cancer 17, 605–619 (2017). https://doi.org/10.1038/nrc.2017.69

64. Pavlov K, Maley CC. New models of neoplastic progression in Barrett's oesophagus. Biochem Soc Trans. 2010;38(2):331-336. doi:10.1042/BST0380331

65. Teles FRF, Alawi F, Castilho RM, Wang Y. Association or causation? Exploring the oral microbiome and cancer links. J Dent Res. 2020 Dec;99(13):1411-1424. doi: 10.1177/0022034520945242. Epub 2020 Aug 18. PMID: 32811287; PMCID: PMC7684840.

66. Seyfried TN, Flores RE, Poff AM, D'Agostino DP. Cancer as a metabolic disease: implications for novel therapeutics.

Carcinogenesis. 2014;35(3):515-527. doi:10.1093/carcin/bgt480

67. Rao VR, Perez-Neut M, Kaja S, Gentile S. Voltage-gated ion channels in cancer cell proliferation. Cancers. 2015;7(2):849-875. doi:10.3390/cancers7020813

68. Chatterjee A, Rodger EJ, Eccles MR. Epigenetic drivers of tumourigenesis and cancer metastasis. Seminars in Cancer Biology. 2018;51:149-159. doi:10.1016/j.semcancer.2017.08.004

69. Theodor Boveri. Concerning the Origin of Malignant Tumours. Company Of Biologists ; Woodbury, N.Y; 2008.

70. Sonnenschein C, Soto AM. Over a century of cancer research: Inconvenient truths and promising leads. PLOS Biology. 2020;18(4):e3000670. doi:10.1371/journal.pbio.3000670

71. Miller WB, Torday JS. A systematic approach to cancer: evolution beyond selection. Clinical and Translational Medicine. 2017;6(1):2. doi:10.1186/s40169-016-0131-4

72. Laconi E, Marongiu F, DeGregori J. Cancer as a disease of old age: changing mutational and microenvironmental landscapes. Br J Cancer 122, 943–952 (2020). https://doi.org/10.1038/s41416-019-0721-1

73. Birkbak NJ, McGranahan N. Cancer genome evolutionary trajectories in metastasis. Cancer Cell. 2020;37(1):8-19. doi:10.1016/j.ccell.2019.12.004

74. Edelman LB, Eddy JA, Price ND. In silico models of cancer. Wiley Interdiscip Rev Syst Biol Med. 2010 Jul-Aug;2(4):438-459. doi: 10.1002/wsbm.75. PMID: 20836040; PMCID: PMC3157287.

75. Bussey KJ, Davies PCW. Reverting to single-cell biology: The predictions of the atavism theory of cancer. Prog

Biophys Mol Biol. 2021 Oct;165:49-55. doi: 10.1016/j.pbiomolbio.2021.08.002. Epub 2021 Aug 8. PMID: 34371024.

76. Deisboeck TS, Couzin ID. Collective behavior in cancer cell populations. BioEssays. 2009;31(2):190-197. doi:10.1002/bies.200800084

77. Alberts B, Johnson A, Lewis J, et al. Molecular Biology of the Cell. 4th edition. New York: Garland Science; 2002. The molecular basis of cancer-cell behavior. Available from: https://www.ncbi.nlm.nih.gov/books/NBK26902/

78. Fang Y, Wang L, Wan C, Sun Y, Van der Jeught K, Zhou Z, Dong T, So KM, Yu T, Li Y, Eyvani H, Colter AB, Dong E, Cao S, Wang J, Schneider BP, Sandusky GE, Liu Y, Zhang C, Lu X, Zhang X. MAL2 drives immune evasion in breast cancer by suppressing tumor antigen presentation. J Clin Invest. 2021 Jan 4;131(1):e140837. doi: 10.1172/JCI140837. PMID: 32990678; PMCID: PMC7773365.

79. Missiroli S, Perrone M, Genovese I, Pinton P, Giorgi C. Cancer metabolism and mitochondria: Finding novel mechanisms to fight tumours. EBioMedicine. 2020;59:102943. doi:10.1016/j.ebiom.2020.102943

80. Claypool SM, Koehler CM. The complexity of cardiolipin in health and disease. Trends Biochem Sci. 2012;37(1):32-41. doi:10.1016/j.tibs.2011.09.003

81. Alfarouk KO, Verduzco D, Rauch C, Muddathir AK, Adil HB, Elhassan GO, et al. Glycolysis, tumor metabolism, cancer growth and dissemination. A new pH-based etiopathogenic perspective and therapeutic approach to an old cancer question. Oncoscience. 2014;1(12):777

82. Maley, C. C. et al. Classifying the evolutionary and ecological features of neoplasms. Nat. Rev. Cancer 17, 605–619 (2017).

83. Gonzalez H, Hagerling C, Werb Z. Roles of the immune system in cancer: from tumor initiation to metastatic progression. Genes & Development. 2018;32(19-20):1267-1284. doi:10.1101/gad.314617.118

84. Ribatti D, Mangialardi G, Vacca A. Stephen Paget and the 'seed and soil' theory of metastatic dissemination. Clin Exp Med. 2006 Dec;6(4):145-9. doi: 10.1007/s10238-006-0117-4. PMID: 17191105.

85. National cancer institute. Metastatic Cancer. National Cancer Institute. Published 2015. https://www.cancer.gov/types/metastatic-cancer

86. Zhang H, Freitas D, Kim HS, et al. Identification of distinct nanoparticles and subsets of extracellular vesicles by asymmetric flow field-flow fractionation. Nat Cell Biol. 2018;20(3):332-343. doi:10.1038/s41556-018-0040-4

87. Ribeiro M, Elghajiji A, Fraser SP, Burke ZD, Tosh D, Djamgoz MBA, Rocha PRF. Human breast cancer cells demonstrate electrical excitability. Front Neurosci. 2020 Apr 30;14:404. doi: 10.3389/fnins.2020.00404. PMID: 32425751; PMCID: PMC7204841.

88. Trigos AS, Pearson RB, Papenfuss AT, Goode DL. How the evolution of multicellularity set the stage for cancer. Br J Cancer. 2018;118(2):145-152. doi:10.1038/bjc.2017.398

89. Marusyk A, Polyak K. Tumor heterogeneity: causes and consequences. Biochim Biophys Acta. 2010;1805(1):105-117. doi:10.1016/j.bbcan.2009.11.002

90. Amend SR, Pienta KJ. Ecology meets cancer biology: the cancer swamp promotes the lethal cancer phenotype. Oncotarget. 2015;6(12):9669-9678. doi:10.18632/oncotarget.3430

91. Ponomarev AV, Shubina IZ. Insights into mechanisms of tumor and immune system interaction: association with

wound healing. Front Oncol. 2019;9:1115. Published 2019 Oct 25. doi:10.3389/fonc.2019.01115

92. Nunes FD, de Almeida FC, Tucci R, de Sousa SC. Homeobox genes: a molecular link between development and cancer. Pesqui Odontol Bras. 2003 Jan-Mar;17(1):94-8. doi: 10.1590/s1517-74912003000100018. Epub 2003 Aug 5. PMID: 12908068.

93. Pelengaris, S., Khan, M. & Evan, G. c-MYC: more than just a matter of life and death. Nat Rev Cancer 2, 764–776 (2002). https://doi.org/10.1038/nrc904

94. Martone R. Scientists discover children's cells living in mothers' brains. Scientific American. https://www.scientificamerican.com/article/scientists-discover-childrens-cells-living-in-mothers-brain/

95. Cells form into "xenobots" on their own. Quanta Magazine. https://www.quantamagazine.org/cells-form-into-xenobots-on-their-own-20210331/

96. Do human "tails" represent the simple "turning on" of genes retained from our ancestors? Evolution News. Published May 13, 2014. Accessed December 8, 2021. https://evolutionnews.org/2014/05/do_human_tails_/

97. Lineweaver CH, Bussey KJ, Blackburn AC, Davies PCW. Cancer progression as a sequence of atavistic reversions. BioEssays. 2021;43(7):2000305. doi:10.1002/bies.202000305

98. Bussey KJ, Davies PCW. Reverting to single-cell biology: the predictions of the atavism theory of cancer. Progress in Biophysics and Molecular Biology. 2021;165:49-55. doi:10.1016/j.pbiomolbio.2021.08.002

99. Cisneros LH, Vaske C, Bussey KJ. Identification of a signature of evolutionarily conserved stress-induced mutagenesis in cancer. bioRxiv. Published April 17, 2021

Accessed December 8, 2021. https://www.biorxiv.org/content/10.1101/2021.04.17.440291v2.full

100. Chernet B, Levin M. Endogenous voltage potentials and the microenvironment: bioelectric signals that reveal, induce and normalize cancer. J Clin Exp Oncol. 2013;Suppl 1:S1-002. doi:10.4172/2324-9110.S1-002

101. Warburg O. On the Origin of Cancer Cells. Science. 1956;123(3191):309-314. doi:10.1126/science.123.3191.309

102. Levine AJ, Jenkins NA, Copeland NG. The roles of initiating truncal mutations in human cancers: the order of mutations and tumor cell type matters. Cancer Cell. 2019;35(1):10-15. doi:10.1016/j.ccell.2018.11.009

103. What is a second cancer? Cancer.net. Published September 12, 2018. Accessed December 9, 2021. https://www.cancer.net/survivorship/what-second-cancer

104. Soto AM, Sonnenschein C. The tissue organization field theory of cancer: a testable replacement for the somatic mutation theory. Bioessays. 2011;33(5):332-340. doi:10.1002/bies.201100025

105. Djamgoz MBA, Fraser SP, Brackenbury WJ. In vivo evidence for voltage-gated sodium channel expression in carcinomas and potentiation of metastasis. Cancers. 2019;11(11):1675. doi:10.3390/cancers11111675

106. Taichman RS, Cooper C, Keller ET, Pienta KJ, Taichman NS, McCauley LK. Use of the stromal cell-derived factor-1/CXCR4 pathway in prostate cancer metastasis to bone. Cancer Research. 2002;62(6):1832-1837. Accessed December 9, 2021. https://pubmed.ncbi.nlm.nih.gov/11912162/

107. Archetti M. Cooperation between cancer cells. Evol Med Public Health. 2018;2018(1):1. Published 2018 Jan 23. doi:10.1093/emph/eoy003

108. Ungefroren H, Sebens S, Seidl D, Lehnert H, Hass R. Interaction of tumor cells with the microenvironment. Cell Commun Signal. 2011;9:18. Published 2011 Sep 13. doi:10.1186/1478-811X-9-18

109. Parker TM, Gupta K, Palma AM, et al. Cell competition in intratumoral and tumor microenvironment interactions. The EMBO journal. 2021;40(17):e107271. doi:10.15252/embj.2020107271

110. Levin M. The computational boundary of a "self": developmental bioelectricity drives multicellularity and scale-free cognition. Front Psychol. 2019;10:2688. Published 2019 Dec 13. doi:10.3389/fpsyg.2019.02688

111. Chahar HS, Bao X, Casola A. Exosomes and their role in the life cycle and pathogenesis of RNA viruses. Viruses. 2015;7(6):3204-3225. Published 2015 Jun 19. doi:10.3390/v7062770

112. Wortzel I, Dror S, Kenific CM, Lyden D. Exosome-mediated metastasis: communication from a distance. Developmental Cell. 2019;49(3):347-360. doi:10.1016/j.devcel.2019.04.011

113. Ledford H. Cancer cells can "infect" normal neighbours. Nature. Published online October 23, 2014. doi:10.1038/nature.2014.16212

114. Peeters CFJM, Geus L-F de, Westphal JR, et al. Decrease in circulating anti-angiogenic factors (angiostatin and endostatin) after surgical removal of primary colorectal carcinoma coincides with increased metabolic activity of liver metastases. Surgery. 2005;137(2):246-249. doi:10.1016/j.surg.2004.06.004

115. Kaukonen R, Mai A, Georgiadou M, et al. Normal stroma suppresses cancer cell proliferation via mechanosensitive regulation of JMJD1a-mediated transcription. Nature Communications. 2016;7(1):12237. doi:10.1038/ncomms12237

116. Théry C, Witwer KW, Aikawa E, et al. Minimal information for studies of extracellular vesicles 2018 (MISEV2018): a position statement of the International Society for Extracellular Vesicles and update of the MISEV2014 guidelines. Journal of Extracellular Vesicles. 2018;7(1):1535750. doi:10.1080/20013078.2018.1535750

117. Shaashua L, Eckerling A, Israeli B, et al. Spontaneous regression of micro-metastases following primary tumor excision: a critical role for primary tumor secretome. BMC Biology. 2020;18(1). doi:10.1186/s12915-020-00893-2

118. Mohr SJ, Whitesel JA. Spontaneous regression of renal cell carcinoma metastases after preoperative embolization of primary tumor and subsequent nephrectomy. Urology. 1979;14(1):5-8. doi:10.1016/0090-4295(79)90201-2

119. Doglioni G, Parik S, Fendt SM. Interactions in the (pre)metastatic niche support metastasis formation. Front Oncol. 2019;9:219. Published 2019 Apr 24. doi:10.3389/fonc.2019.00219

120. What Is a Cancer of Unknown Primary? www.cancer.org. Accessed December 10, 2021. https://www.cancer.org/cancer/cancer-unknown-primary/about/cancer-of-unknown-primary.html

121. Dhatchinamoorthy K, Colbert JD, Rock KL. Cancer immune evasion through loss of MHC class I antigen presentation. Front Immunol. 2021;12:636568. Published 2021 Mar 9. doi:10.3389/fimmu.2021.636568

122. Lin Y, Xu J, Lan H. Tumor-associated macrophages in tumor metastasis: biological roles and clinical therapeutic

applications. Journal of Hematology & Oncology. 2019;12(1). doi:10.1186/s13045-019-0760-3

123. Huang R, Wang S, Wang N, et al. CCL5 derived from tumor-associated macrophages promotes prostate cancer stem cells and metastasis via activating β-catenin/STAT3 signaling. Cell Death & Disease. 2020;11(4):1-20. doi:10.1038/s41419-020-2435-y

124. Croft NP, Smith SA, Pickering J, et al. Most viral peptides displayed by class I MHC on infected cells are immunogenic. Proceedings of the National Academy of Sciences. 2019;116(8):3112-3117. doi:10.1073/pnas.1815239116

125. Facciabene A, Motz GT, Coukos G. T-regulatory cells: key players in tumor immune escape and angiogenesis. Cancer Res. 2012;72(9):2162-2171. doi:10.1158/0008-5472.CAN-11-3687

126. Lu B, Finn OJ. T-cell death and cancer immune tolerance. Cell Death & Differentiation. 2007;15(1):70-79. doi:10.1038/sj.cdd.4402274

127. Cochran AJ, Morton DL, Stern S, Lana AMA, Essner R, Wen D-R. Sentinel lymph nodes show profound downregulation of antigen-presenting cells of the paracortex: implications for tumor biology and treatment. Modern Pathology. 2001;14(6):604-608. doi:10.1038/modpathol.3880358

128. Krishna S, Lowery FJ, Copeland AR, et al. Stem-like CD8 T cells mediate response of adoptive cell immunotherapy against human cancer. Science. 2020;370(6522):1328-1334. doi:10.1126/science.abb9847

129. Yuen GJ, Demissie E, Pillai S. B lymphocytes and cancer: a love-hate relationship. Trends Cancer. 2016;2(12):747-757. doi:10.1016/j.trecan.2016.10.010

130. Kleef R, Hager ED. Fever, pyrogens and cancer. Landes Bioscience; 2013. Accessed December 10, 2021. https://www.ncbi.nlm.nih.gov/books/NBK6084/

131. Astigiano S, Damonte P, Fossati S, Boni L, Barbieri O. Fate of embryonal carcinoma cells injected into postimplantation mouse embryos. Differentiation; Research in Biological Diversity. 2005;73(9-10):484-490. doi:10.1111/j.1432-0436.2005.00043.x

132. Chernet BT, Adams DS, Lobikin M, Levin M. Use of genetically encoded, light-gated ion translocators to control tumorigenesis. Oncotarget. 2016;7(15):19575-19588. doi:10.18632/oncotarget.8036

133. Brodeur GM. Spontaneous regression of neuroblastoma. Cell Tissue Res. 2018;372(2):277-286. doi:10.1007/s00441-017-2761-2

134. Zheng J, Gao P. Toward normalization of the tumor microenvironment for cancer therapy. Integr Cancer Ther. 2019;18:1534735419862352. doi:10.1177/1534735419862352

135. Maffini MV, Calabro JM, Soto AM, Sonnenschein C. Stromal regulation of neoplastic development: age-dependent normalization of neoplastic mammary cells by mammary stroma. American Journal of Pathology. 2005;167:1405–10. 10.1016/S0002-9440(10)61227-8

136. Ambros IM, Zellner A, Roald B, Amann G, Ladenstein R, Printz D, et al. Role of ploidy, chromosome 1p, and Schwann cells in the maturation of neuroblastoma. N Engl J Med. 1996;334(23):1505–11. Epub 1996/06/06. 10.1056/NEJM199606063342304

137. Genua F, Raghunathan V, Jenab M, Gallagher WM, Hughes DJ. The role of gut barrier dysfunction and microbiome dysbiosis in colorectal cancer development. Front Oncol.

2021;11:626349. Published 2021 Apr 15. doi:10.3389/fonc.2021.626349

138. Marsman WA, Westerterp M, van Heek NJ, ten Kate FJ, Izbicki JR, van Lanschot JJ. Epithelial cells in bone marrow: do they matter?. Gut. 2005;54(12):1821-1822. doi:10.1136/gut.2005.078774

139. Micrometastasis - an overview | ScienceDirect Topics. www.sciencedirect.com. Accessed December 11, 2021. https://www.sciencedirect.com/topics/medicine-and-dentistry/micrometastasis

140. Strand therapeutics' mRNA logic circuits enhance gene therapy's safety, ease and controllability. BioSpace. Accessed December 11, 2021. https://www.biospace.com/article/strand-therapeutics-mrna-logic-circuits-enhance-gene-therapy-s-safety-ease-and-controllability-/

141. Moresco EM, Li X, Beutler B. Going forward with genetics: recent technological advances and forward genetics in mice. Am J Pathol. 2013;182(5):1462-1473. doi:10.1016/j.ajpath.2013.02.002

142. Why do researchers investigate zebrafish? www.mpg.de. Accessed December 11, 2021. https://www.mpg.de/10973793/why-do-scientists-investigate-zebra-fish

143. Samuel Sidi, PhD. Pershing Square Foundation. Accessed December 11, 2021. https://psscra.org/winners/samuel-sidi-phd/

144. Liu PH, Shah RB, Li Y, et al. An IRAK1–PIN1 signalling axis drives intrinsic tumour resistance to radiation therapy. Nature Cell Biology. 2019;21(2):203-213. doi:10.1038/s41556-018-0260-7

145. Ruiz-Delgado GJ, Nuñez-Cortez AK, Olivares-Gazca JC, Fortiz YC, Ruiz-Argüelles A, Ruiz-Argüelles GJ. Lineage switch from acute lymphoblastic leukemia to myeloid leukemia. Medicina Universitaria. 2017;19(74):27-31. doi:10.1016/j.rmu.2017.02.001

146. Gupta K, Gupta S. Neuroendocrine differentiation in prostate cancer: key epigenetic players. Transl Cancer Res. 2017;6(Suppl 1):S104-S108. doi:10.21037/tcr.2017.01.20

147. Deshmukh AP, Vasaikar SV, Tomczak K, et al. Identification of EMT signaling cross-talk and gene regulatory networks by single-cell RNA sequencing. Proceedings of the National Academy of Sciences of the United States of America. 2021;118(19):e2102050118. doi:10.1073/pnas.2102050118

148. Tan WCC, Nerurkar SN, Cai HY, et al. Overview of multiplex immunohistochemistry/immunofluorescence techniques in the era of cancer immunotherapy. Cancer Commun (Lond). 2020;40(4):135-153. doi:10.1002/cac2.12023

149. Yin J, Valin KL, Dixon ML, Leavenworth JW. The role of microglia and macrophages in CNS homeostasis, autoimmunity, and cancer. Journal of Immunology Research. 2017;2017:1-12. doi:10.1155/2017/5150678

150. Casanova-Acebes M, Dalla E, Leader AM, et al. Tissue-resident macrophages provide a pro-tumorigenic niche to early NSCLC cells. Nature. 2021;595(7868):578-584. doi:10.1038/s41586-021-03651-8

151. Yao J, Ly D, Dervovic D, et al. Human double negative T cells target lung cancer via ligand-dependent mechanisms that can be enhanced by IL-15. Journal for ImmunoTherapy of Cancer. 2019;7(1). doi:10.1186/s40425-019-0507-2

152. Lee J, Minden MD, Chen WC, et al. Allogeneic human double negative T cells as a novel immunotherapy for acute

myeloid leukemia and its underlying mechanisms. Clinical Cancer Research. 2018;24(2):370-382. doi:10.1158/1078-0432.CCR-17-2228

153. Roser M, Ritchie H. Cancer. Our World in Data. Published July 2015. https://ourworldindata.org/cancer

154. The naked eye alone is not enough to ensure the accurate diagnosis of skin cancer, say experts. ScienceDaily. Accessed December 12, 2021. https://www.sciencedaily.com/releases/2018/12/181207210800.htm

155. What is a Tyrer-Cuzick score and what do the results mean? www.medicalnewstoday.com. Published September 22, 2021. Accessed December 12, 2021. https://www.medicalnewstoday.com/articles/tyrer-cuzick-score#scoring-factors

156. BreastCancer.org. U.S. Breast Cancer Statistics | Breastcancer.org. Breastcancer.org. Published June 25, 2020. https://www.breastcancer.org/symptoms/understand_bc/statistics

157. Løberg M, Lousdal ML, Bretthauer M, Kalager M. Benefits and harms of mammography screening. Breast Cancer Res. 2015;17(1):63. Published 2015 May 1. doi:10.1186/s13058-015-0525-z

158. Hofman V, Heeke S, Allègra M, Ilié M, Hofman P. Liquid Biopsy and Genomic Assessment for Lung Cancer. Published 2019. Accessed December 12, 2021. https://www.sciencedirect.com/topics/medicine-and-dentistry/liquid-biopsy

159. Kilgour E, Rothwell DG, Brady G, Dive C. Liquid biopsy-based biomarkers of treatment response and resistance. Cancer Cell. 2020;37(4):485-495. doi:10.1016/j.ccell.2020.03.012

160. Malik A, Srinivasan S, Batra J. A new era of prostate cancer precision medicine. Front Oncol. 2019;9:1263. Published 2019 Nov 26. doi:10.3389/fonc.2019.01263

161. Shyamala K, Girish HC, Murgod S. Risk of tumor cell seeding through biopsy and aspiration cytology. J Int Soc Prev Community Dent. 2014;4(1):5-11. doi:10.4103/2231-0762.129446

162. Biopsy - Better Health Channel. www.betterhealth.vic.gov.au. Accessed December 12, 2021. https://www.betterhealth.vic.gov.au/health/conditionsandtreatments/biopsy#complications-from-a-biopsy

163. Willis CM, Church SM, Guest CM, et al. Olfactory detection of human bladder cancer by dogs: proof of principle study. BMJ. 2004;329(7468):712. doi:10.1136/bmj.329.7468.712

164. How this dog saved its owner's life by warning her she'd breast cancer. belfasttelegraph. https://www.belfasttelegraph.co.uk/life/features/how-this-dog-saved-its-owners-life-by-warning-her-shed-breast-cancer-30215823.html. Accessed December 12, 2021.

165. Guest C, Harris R, Sfanos KS, et al. Feasibility of integrating canine olfaction with chemical and microbial profiling of urine to detect lethal prostate cancer. Culig Z, ed. PLOS ONE. 2021;16(2):e0245530. doi:10.1371/journal.pone.0245530

166. Tucker I. Diseases that dogs can detect. The Guardian. https://www.theguardian.com/technology/2018/nov/04/five-diseases-that-dogs-can-detect. Published November 4, 2018.

167. Toward a disease-sniffing device that rivals a dog's nose. MIT News | Massachusetts Institute of Technology. https://news.mit.edu/2021/disease-detection-device-dogs-0217

168. Liu F, Xu X, Zhu H, et al. PET Imaging of 18F-(2 S,4 R)4-fluoroglutamine accumulation in breast cancer: from xenografts to patients. Molecular Pharmaceutics. 2018;15(8):3448-3455. doi:10.1021/acs.molpharmaceut.8b00430

169. Almuhaideb A, Papathanasiou N, Bomanji J. 18 F-FDG PET/CT Imaging in oncology. Annals of Saudi Medicine. 2011;31(1):3-13. doi:10.4103/0256-4947.75771

170. Fischer BM, Olsen MWB, Ley CD, et al. How few cancer cells can be detected by positron emission tomography? A frequent question addressed by an in vitro study. European Journal of Nuclear Medicine and Molecular Imaging. 2006;33(6):697-702. doi:10.1007/s00259-005-0038-6

171. The Circulating Cell-free Genome Atlas Study - full text view - ClinicalTrials.gov. Clinicaltrials.gov. Published 2020. https://clinicaltrials.gov/ct2/show/NCT02889978

172. GRAIL announces first health system to offer Galleri, novel multi-cancer early detection blood test. GRAIL. Accessed December 12, 2021. https://grail.com/press-releases/grail-announces-first-health-system-to-offer-galleri-novel-multi-cancer-early-detection-blood-test/

173. Hubbell E, Clarke CA, Aravanis AM, Berg CD. Modeled reductions in late-stage cancer with a multi-cancer early detection test. Cancer Epidemiology and Prevention Biomarkers. 2021;30(3):460-468. doi:10.1158/1055-9965.EPI-20-1134

174. Nadauld LD, McDonnell CH 3rd, Beer TM, et al. The PATHFINDER study: assessment of the implementation of an investigational multi-cancer early detection test into clinical practice. Cancers (Basel). 2021;13(14):3501. Published 2021 Jul 13. doi:10.3390/cancers13143501

175. Horst C, Dickson J, Tisi S, et al. P41.04 The SUMMIT study: pulmonary nodule and incidental findings in the first

10,000 participants of a population-based low-dose CT screening study. Journal of Thoracic Oncology. 2021;16(3):S473-S474. doi:10.1016/j.jtho.2021.01.818

176. Ballard-Barbash R, Friedenreich CM, Courneya KS, Siddiqi SM, McTiernan A, Alfano CM. Physical Activity, biomarkers, and disease outcomes in cancer survivors: a systematic review. JNCI Journal of the National Cancer Institute. 2012;104(11):815-840. doi:10.1093/jnci/djs207

177. Three-drug combination found most effective in treating HIV infection. news.stanford.edu. Accessed December 13, 2021. https://news.stanford.edu/news/2004/january14/aids.html

178. Delbaldo C, Michiels S, Syz N, Soria J-C, Le Chevalier T, Pignon J-P. Benefits of Adding a Drug to a Single-Agent or a 2-Agent Chemotherapy Regimen in Advanced Non–Small-Cell Lung CancerA Meta-analysis. JAMA. 2004;292(4):470-484. doi:10.1001/jama.292.4.470

179. Janku F. Tumor heterogeneity in the clinic: is it a real problem? Ther Adv Med Oncol. 2014;6(2):43-51. doi:10.1177/1758834013517414

180. Biopsy technique - an overview | ScienceDirect Topics. www.sciencedirect.com. Accessed December 13, 2021. https://www.sciencedirect.com/topics/medicine-and-dentistry/biopsy-technique

181. Zitvogel L, Apetoh L, Ghiringhelli F, Kroemer G. Immunological aspects of cancer chemotherapy. Nature Reviews Immunology. 2008;8(1):59-73. doi:10.1038/nri2216

182. Liu J-W, Chen C, Loh E-W, et al. Tyrosine kinase inhibitors for advanced or metastatic thyroid cancer: a meta-analysis of randomized controlled trials. Current Medical Research and Opinion. 2018;34(5):795-803. doi:10.1080/03007995.2017.1368466

183. Janiszewska M, Stein S, Filho OM, et al. The impact of tumor epithelial and microenvironmental heterogeneity on treatment responses in HER2+ breast cancer. JCI Insight. 2021;6(11). doi:10.1172/jci.insight.147617

184. Pienta KJ, Hammarlund EU, Axelrod R, Brown JS, Amend SR. Poly-aneuploid cancer cells promote evolvability, generating lethal cancer. Evolutionary Applications. 2020;13(7):1626-1634. doi:10.1111/eva.12929

185. Kostecka LG, Pienta KJ, Amend SR. Polyaneuploid cancer cell dormancy: lessons from evolutionary phyla. Frontiers in Ecology and Evolution. 2021;9:660755. doi:10.3389/fevo.2021.660755

186. Aboalela N, Lyon D, Elswick RK, et al. Perceived stress levels, chemotherapy, radiation treatment and tumor characteristics are associated with a persistent increased frequency of somatic chromosomal instability in women diagnosed with breast cancer: a one year longitudinal study. Sung S-Y, ed. PLOS ONE. 2015;10(7):e0133380. doi:10.1371/journal.pone.0133380

187. National Cancer Institute. Immune checkpoint inhibitors. National Cancer Institute. Published September 24, 2019. https://www.cancer.gov/about-cancer/treatment/types/immunotherapy/checkpoint-inhibitors

188. Rotte A. Combination of CTLA-4 and PD-1 blockers for treatment of cancer. Journal of Experimental & Clinical Cancer Research. 2019;38(1). doi:10.1186/s13046-019-1259-z

189. Wollmann G, Rogulin V, Simon I, Rose JK, van den Pol AN. Some attenuated variants of vesicular stomatitis virus show enhanced oncolytic activity against human glioblastoma cells relative to normal brain cells. J Virol. 2010;84(3):1563-1573. doi:10.1128/JVI.02040-09

190. Neoadjuvant chemotherapy prior to surgery holds benefit in pancreatic cancer. Targeted Oncology. Accessed December 13, 2021. https://www.targetedonc.com/view/neoadjuvant-chemotherapy-prior-to-surgery-holds-benefit-in-pancreatic-cancer

191. Topalian SL, Taube JM, Pardoll DM. Neoadjuvant checkpoint blockade for cancer immunotherapy. Science. 2020;367(6477). doi:10.1126/science.aax0182

192. Prasad V, Kaestner V. Nivolumab and pembrolizumab: monoclonal antibodies against programmed cell death-1 (PD-1) that are interchangeable. Seminars in Oncology. 2017;44(2):132-135. doi:10.1053/j.seminoncol.2017.06.007

193. Ralli M, Botticelli A, Visconti IC, et al. Immunotherapy in the treatment of metastatic melanoma: current knowledge and future directions. Journal of Immunology Research. 2020;2020:1-12. doi:10.1155/2020/9235638

194. Seyfried TN, Shivane AG, Kalamian M, Maroon JC, Mukherjee P, Zuccoli G. Ketogenic metabolic therapy, without chemo or radiation, for the long-term management of IDH1-mutant glioblastoma: an 80-month follow-up case report. Front Nutr. 2021;8:682243. Published 2021 May 31. doi:10.3389/fnut.2021.682243

195. Iyikesici MS, Slocum S, Turkmen E, Akdemir O, Slocum AK, Berkarda FB. Complete response of locally advanced (stage III) rectal Cancer to metabolically supported chemoradiotherapy with hyperthermia. International Journal of Cancer Research and Molecular Mechanisms ( ISSN 2381-3318 ). 2016;2(1). doi:10.16966/2381-3318.120

196. Jing X, Yang F, Shao C, et al. Role of hypoxia in cancer therapy by regulating the tumor microenvironment. Molecular Cancer. 2019;18(1). doi:10.1186/s12943-019-1089-9

197. Graham K, Unger E. Overcoming tumor hypoxia as a barrier to radiotherapy, chemotherapy and immunotherapy in cancer treatment. International Journal of Nanomedicine. 2018;Volume 13:6049-6058. doi:10.2147/ijn.s140462

198. Teicher BA. Hypoxia and drug resistance. Cancer and Metastasis Reviews. 1994;13(2):139-168. doi:10.1007/bf00689633

199. Ohguri T, Kunugita N, Yahara K, et al. Efficacy of hyperbaric oxygen therapy combined with mild hyperthermia for improving the anti-tumour effects of carboplatin. International Journal of Hyperthermia. 2015;31(6):643-648. doi:10.3109/02656736.2015.1055832

200. İyikesici MS, Slocum AK, Winters N, Kalamian M, Seyfried TN. Metabolically supported chemotherapy for managing end-stage breast cancer: a complete and durable response. Cureus. Published online April 26, 2021. doi:10.7759/cureus.14686

201. Iyikesici M. Long-term survival outcomes of metabolically supported chemotherapy with gemcitabine-based or FOLFIRINOX regimen combined with ketogenic diet, hyperthermia, and hyperbaric oxygen therapy in metastatic pancreatic cancer. Complementary Medicine Research. 2019;27(1):31-39. doi:10.1159/000502135

202. İyikesici MS, Slocum AK, Slocum A, Berkarda FB, Kalamian M, Seyfried TN. Efficacy of metabolically supported chemotherapy combined with ketogenic diet, hyperthermia, and hyperbaric oxygen therapy for stage IV triple-negative breast cancer. Cureus. Published online July 7, 2017. doi:10.7759/cureus.1445

203. Iyikesici MS. Feasibility study of metabolically supported chemotherapy with weekly carboplatin/paclitaxel combined with ketogenic diet, hyperthermia and hyperbaric oxygen therapy in metastatic non-small cell lung cancer.

International Journal of Hyperthermia. 2019;36(1):445-454. doi:10.1080/02656736.2019.1589584

204. Yokouchi. Hyperbaric oxygen as a chemotherapy adjuvant in the treatment of osteosarcoma. Oncology Reports. 2009;22(05). doi:10.3892/or_00000534

205. Suzuki Y, Tanaka K, Negishi D, et al. Pharmacokinetic investigation of increased efficacy against malignant gliomas of carboplatin combined with hyperbaric oxygenation. Neurologia Medico-Chirurgica. 2009;49(5):193-197; discussion 197. doi:10.2176/nmc.49.193

206. Jain KK. Textbook of Hyperbaric Medicine. Role of HBO in enhancing cancer radiosensitivity. Published online 2017:523-531. doi:10.1007/978-3-319-47140-2_38

207. Hofmann P. Cancer and exercise: Warburg hypothesis, tumour metabolism and high-intensity anaerobic exercise. Sports. 2018;6(1):10. doi:10.3390/sports6010010

208. Olgun A. Biological effects of deuteronation: ATP synthase as an example. Theoretical Biology and Medical Modelling. 2007;4(1). doi:10.1186/1742-4682-4-9

209. Mendoza-Hoffmann F, Zarco-Zavala M, Ortega R, García-Trejo JJ. Control of rotation of the F1FO-ATP synthase nanomotor by an inhibitory α-helix from unfolded ε or intrinsically disordered ζ and IF1 proteins. Journal of Bioenergetics and Biomembranes. 2018;50(5):403-424. doi:10.1007/s10863-018-9773-9

210. Urbauer JL, Dorgan LJ, Schuster SM. Effects of deuterium on the kinetics of beef heart mitochondrial ATPase. Archives of Biochemistry and Biophysics. 1984;231(2):498-502. doi:10.1016/0003-9861(84)90413-2

211. Boros L. Biological nanomechanics: ATP synthesis and deuterium depletion. Lecture presented at: Los Angeles Biomedical Research Institute at the Harbor-UCLA Medical

Center - Liu Research Building; August 2016; Los Angeles, CA.

212. Veech RL, Valeri CR. Using D-ß-hydroxybutyrate containing solutions to treat hyperglycemia induced by shock or injury instead of Insulin may circumvent insulin resistance and provide cells with the energy required to maintain vital processes through preserving normal mitochondrial function without causing hypoglycemia. clinmedjournalsorg. Accessed December 14, 2021. https://clinmedjournals.org/articles/tcr/trauma-cases-and-reviews-tcr-2-025.php?jid=tcr

213. Abdelwahab MG, Fenton KE, Preul MC, et al. The ketogenic diet is an effective adjuvant to radiation therapy for the treatment of malignant glioma. PLoS One. 2012;7(5):e36197. doi:10.1371/journal.pone.0036197

214. Klement RJ, Champ CE. Calories, carbohydrates, and cancer therapy with radiation: exploiting the five R's through dietary manipulation. Cancer and Metastasis Reviews. 2014;33(1):217-229. doi:10.1007/s10555-014-9495-3

215. Poff AM, Ari C, Arnold P, Seyfried TN, D'Agostino DP. Ketone supplementation decreases tumor cell viability and prolongs survival of mice with metastatic cancer. Int J Cancer. 2014;135(7):1711-1720. doi:10.1002/ijc.28809

216. Cannioto RA, Hutson A, Dighe S, et al. Physical activity before, during, and after chemotherapy for high-risk breast cancer: relationships with survival. JNCI: Journal of the National Cancer Institute. Published online April 2, 2020. doi:10.1093/jnci/djaa046

217. Azrad M, Demark-Wahnefried W. The association between adiposity and breast cancer recurrence and survival: A review of the recent literature. Curr Nutr Rep. 2014;3(1):9-15. doi:10.1007/s13668-013-0068-9

218. Burke L, Guterman I, Palacios Gallego R, et al. The Janus-like role of proline metabolism in cancer. Cell Death Discovery. 2020;6(1). doi:10.1038/s41420-020-00341-8

219. Mukherjee PK, Funchain P, Retuerto M, et al. Metabolomic analysis identifies differentially produced oral metabolites, including the oncometabolite 2-hydroxyglutarate, in patients with head and neck squamous cell carcinoma. BBA Clin. 2016;7:8-15. Published 2016 Dec 18. doi:10.1016/j.bbacli.2016.12.001

220. Berg J. A paradigm shift in glioblastoma treatment and research: a multi-mechanistic, multi-agent approach to target glioblastoma multiforme. Journal of Advanced Medical Sciences and Applied Technologies. 2017;2(4):323. doi:10.18869/nrip.jamsat.2.4.323

221. Cheng WY, Wu C-Y, Yu J. The role of gut microbiota in cancer treatment: friend or foe? Gut. 2020;69(10):1867-1876. doi:10.1136/gutjnl-2020-321153

222. Benler S, Yutin N, Antipov D, et al. Thousands of previously unknown phages discovered in whole-community human gut metagenomes. Microbiome. 2021;9(1). doi:10.1186/s40168-021-01017-w

223. Przerwa A, Zimecki M, Switała-Jeleń K, et al. Effects of bacteriophages on free radical production and phagocytic functions. Medical Microbiology and Immunology. 2006;195(3):143-150. doi:10.1007/s00430-006-0011-4

224. Liou G-Y, Storz P. Reactive oxygen species in cancer. Free Radical Research. 2010;44(5):479-496. doi:10.3109/10715761003667554

225. Çolakoğlu M, Xue J, Trajkovski M. Bacteriophage prevents alcoholic liver disease. Cell. 2020;180(2):218-220. doi:10.1016/j.cell.2019.12.034

226. Gutiérrez B, Domingo-Calap P. Phage therapy in gastrointestinal diseases. Microorganisms. 2020;8(9):1420. Published 2020 Sep 16. doi:10.3390/microorganisms8091420

227. What termites and cells have in common. www.mpg.de. Accessed December 14, 2021. https://www.mpg.de/what-termites-and-cells-have-in-common

228. Canale SD, Louis DZ, Maio V, et al. The relationship between physician empathy and disease complications. Academic Medicine. 2012;87(9):1243-1249. doi:10.1097/acm.0b013e3182628fbf

229. Fogarty LA, Curbow BA, Wingard JR, McDonnell K, Somerfield MR. Can 40 seconds of compassion reduce patient anxiety? Journal of Clinical Oncology. 1999;17(1):371-371. doi:10.1200/jco.1999.17.1.371

230. Sarinopoulos I, Hesson AM, Gordon C, et al. Patient-centered interviewing is associated with decreased responses to painful stimuli: An initial fMRI study. Patient Education and Counseling. 2013;90(2):220-225. doi:10.1016/j.pec.2012.10.021

231. Rakel DP, Hoeft TJ, Barrett BP, Chewning BA, Craig BM, Niu M. Practitioner empathy and the duration of the common cold. Family Medicine. 2009;41(7):494-501. https://pubmed.ncbi.nlm.nih.gov/19582635/

232. Kelley JM, Kraft-Todd G, Schapira L, Kossowsky J, Riess H. The influence of the patient-clinician relationship on healthcare outcomes: a systematic review and meta-analysis of randomized controlled trials. Timmer A, ed. PLoS ONE. 2014;9(4):e94207. doi:10.1371/journal.pone.0094207

233. Reith TP. Burnout in United States healthcare professionals: a narrative review. Cureus. 2018;10(12):e3681. Published 2018 Dec 4. doi:10.7759/cureus.3681

234. Lipton, BH. Chapter 5: Biology and belief. In: The Biology of Belief: Unleashing the Power of Consciousness, Matter & Miracles. Hay House, Inc.; 2008: 93-114.

235. Basanta D, Gatenby RA, Anderson AR. Exploiting evolution to treat drug resistance: combination therapy and the double bind. Mol Pharm. 2012;9(4):914-921. doi:10.1021/mp200458e

236. Maley CC, Reid BJ, Forrest S. Cancer Prevention Strategies That Address the Evolutionary Dynamics of Neoplastic Cells: Simulating Benign Cell Boosters and Selection for Chemosensitivity. Cancer Epidemiology and Prevention Biomarkers. 2004;13(8):1375-1384. Accessed December 14, 2021. https://cebp.aacrjournals.org/content/13/8/1375

237. Zhang J, Cunningham JJ, Brown JS, Gatenby RA. Integrating evolutionary dynamics into treatment of metastatic castrate-resistant prostate cancer. Nature Communications. 2017;8(1). doi:10.1038/s41467-017-01968-5

238. Stereotactic body radiation therapy for breast cancer: Benefits, challenges and choices. appliedradiationoncology.com. Accessed December 14, 2021. https://appliedradiationoncology.com/articles/stereotactic-body-radiation-therapy-for-breast-cancer-benefits-challenges-and-choices

239. Djamgoz MBA, Fraser SP, Brackenbury WJ. In Vivo Evidence for Voltage-Gated Sodium Channel Expression in Carcinomas and Potentiation of Metastasis. Cancers (Basel). 2019;11(11):1675. Published 2019 Oct 28. doi:10.3390/cancers11111675

240. Fraser SP, Onkal R, Theys M, Bosmans F, Djamgoz MBA. Neonatal Na V 1.5 channels: pharmacological distinctiveness of a cancer-related voltage-gated sodium

channel splice variant. British Journal of Pharmacology. Published online December 2, 2021. doi:10.1111/bph.15668

241. Bugan I, Kucuk S, Karagoz Z, et al. Anti-metastatic effect of ranolazine in an in vivo rat model of prostate cancer, and expression of voltage-gated sodium channel protein in human prostate. Prostate Cancer and Prostatic Diseases. 2019;22(4):569-579. doi:10.1038/s41391-019-0128-3

242. DiGeorgio Arch Dermatol. 2010;146(10):1120-1124

243. Xavier-Júnior et al. Surgical and Experimental Pathology (2019) 2:19

244. McCarthy SW, Palmer AA, Bale PM, et al. Naevus cells in lymph nodes. Pathology. 1974;6:351–358.

245. Gonzàlez-Farré M, Ronen S, Keiser E, Prieto VG, Aung PP. Three Types of Nodal Melanocytic Nevi in Sentinel Lymph Nodes of Patients With Melanoma: Pitfalls, Immunohistochemistry, and a Review of the Literature. Am J Dermatopathol. 2020 Oct;42(10):739-744.

246. BJ Coventry Characterisation of Tumour Infiltrating Lymphocytes in Human Solid Tumours: Using Standard and Video Image Analytic Methods for Cellular Quantitation of Immunostained Cells Flinders University of S. Aust. 1991

247. Coventry BJ Therapeutic vaccination immunomodulation: forming the basis of all cancer immunotherapy. Ther Adv Vaccines Immunother. 2019 Aug 1;7:2515135519862234.

248. Coventry BJ, Henneberg M, (Davies PCW) The Immune System and Responses to Cancer: Coordinated Evolution. REVIEW F1000 2015 (Version 3 2021).

249. Coventry BJ, Ashdown ML, Markovic SN. Immune Therapies for Cancer: Bimodality—The Blind Spot to Clinical Efficacy—Lost in Translation. J Immunother 2011 Volume 34, Number 9. 717.

250. Dorraki M, Fouladzadeh A, Salamon SJ, Allison A, Coventry BJ, Abbott D. On detection of periodicity in C-reactive protein (CRP) levels. Sci Rep. 2018 Aug 10;8(1):11979. doi: 10.1038/s41598-018-30469-8.

251. Dorraki M, Fouladzadeh A, Salamon SJ, Allison A, Coventry BJ, Abbott D. Can C-Reactive Protein (CRP) Time Series Forecasting be Achieved via Deep Learning? IEEE Access 2019: 7 May 59311-20.

252. Coventry BJ Australian Broadcasting Commission - Radio National Science Show interview with Robin Williams April 18th 2010 "Rhythms in the Immune System" http://www.abc.net.au/rn/scienceshow/stories/2010/2871586.htm

253. Rosenberg SA IL-2: The First Effective Immunotherapy for Human Cancer J Immunol 2014; 192:5451-545 http://www.jimmunol.org/content/192/12/5451   doi: 10.4049/jimmunol.1490019

254. Bright R, Coventry BJ, Eardley-Harris N, Briggs N. Clinical Response Rates From Interleukin-2 Therapy for Metastatic Melanoma Over 30 Years' Experience: A Meta-Analysis of 3312 Patients. J Immunother. 2017 Jan;40(1):21-30. PubMed PMID: 27875387.

255. Vétizou M, Pitt JM, Daillère R, Lepage P, Waldschmitt N, Flament C, Rusakiewicz S, Routy B, Roberti MP, Duong CP, Poirier-Colame V, Roux A, Becharef S, Formenti S, Golden E, Cording S, Eberl G, Schlitzer A, Ginhoux F, Mani S, Yamazaki T, Jacquelot N, Enot DP, Bérard M, Nigou J, Opolon P, Eggermont A, Woerther PL, Chachaty E, Chaput N, Robert C, Mateus C, Kroemer G, Raoult D, Boneca IG, Carbonnel F, Chamaillard M, Zitvogel L. Anticancer immunotherapy by CTLA-4 blockade relies on the gut microbiota. Science. 2015 Nov 27;350(6264):1079-84. doi: 10.1126/science.aad1329. Epub 2015 Nov 5. PMID: 26541610; PMCID: PMC4721659.

256. Lamb R etal Antibiotics that target mitochondria effectively eradicate cancer stem cells, across multiple tumor types: Treating cancer like an infectious disease Oncotarget, Vol. 6, No.7

257. Andrew A Almonte, Hareesha Rangarajan, Desmond Yip & Aude M Fahrer How does the gut microbiome influence immune checkpoint blockade therapy? Immunology & Cell Biology 2021; 99: 361–372

258. Coventry BJ, Lilly C, Hersey P, Michele A, Bright R Prolonged Repeated Vaccine Immuno-Chemotherapy Induces Long-Term Clinical Responses and Survival for Advanced Metastatic Melanoma. J Immunother. Cancer 2014 2: 9.

259. Coventry BJ, Baum D, Lilly CA Long-term survival in advanced melanoma patients using repeated therapies: Successive immunomodulation improving the odds? Cancer Manag. Res. 2015 Apr 29;7:93-103.

260. Fraser SP, Onkal R, Theys M, Bosmans F, Djamgoz MBA. Neonatal NaV1.5 channels: pharmacological distinctiveness of a cancer-related voltage-gated sodium channel splice variant. Br J Pharmacol. 2021 Aug 19. doi: 10.1111/bph.15668.

261. Insulin in the Adjuvant Breast Cancer Setting: A Novel Therapeutic Target for Lifestyle and Pharmacologic Interventions? Pamela J. Goodwin, Samuel Lunenfeld Research Institute at Mount Sinai Hospital, University of Toronto, Toronto, Ontario, Canada; Journal of Clinical Oncology, Vol 26, No 6 (February 20), 2008: pp 833-834 833 DOI: 10.1200/JCO.20D07 14 7132

262. Progress in Experimental Tumor Research, Editor: F. Homburger, Cambridge, Mass. Publisher: S. Karger, Basel

263. Cancer as a mitochondrial metabolic disease, Thomas N.Seyfried, Biology Department, Boston College, Chestnut

Hill, MA, USA, http://journal.frontiersin.org/article/10.3389/fcell.2015.00043/abstract

264. Genomic profiling of short- and long-term caloric restriction effects in the liver of aging mice, Shelley X. Cao, Joseph M. Dhahbi, Patricia L. Mote, and Stephen R. Spindler, Department of Biochemistry, University of California, Riverside, CA 92521, Edited by Bruce N. Ames, University of California, Berkeley, CA, and approved July 11, 2001 (received for review June 19, 2001)

265. Calorie Restriction in Biosphere 2: Alterations in Physiologic, Hematologic, Hormonal, and Biochemical Parameters in Humans Restricted for a 2-Year Period; Roy L. Walford, Department of Pathology, the Center for Health Sciences, University of California, Los Angeles. Dennis Mock, San Diego Supercomputer Center, University of California, San Diego. Roy Verdery, D. W. Reynolds Department of Geriatrics, The University of Arkansas for Medical Sciences, Little Rock. Taber MacCallum, Paragon Development Co., Tuscon, Arizona. Journal of Gerontology: BIOLOGICAL SCIENCES 2002, Vol. 57A, No.6, B211-B224

266. Seyfried, T.N.; Chinopoulos, C. Can the Mitochondrial Metabolic Theory Explain Better the Origin and Management of Cancer than Can the Somatic Mutation Theory? Metabolites 2021, 11, 572. https://doi.org/10.3390/metabo11090572

267. https://www.frontiersin.org/articles/10.3389/fcell.2021.676344/full

Made in the USA
Las Vegas, NV
17 January 2022